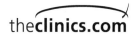

ANESTHESIOLOGY CLINICS

Trauma

GUEST EDITORS
Micha Y. Shamir, MD, and
Yoram G. Weiss, MD

CONSULTING EDITOR
Lee A. Fleisher, MD

March 2007 • Volume 25 • Number 1

SAUNDERS

An Imprint of Elsevier, Inc.
PHILADELPHIA   LONDON   TORONTO   MONTREAL   SYDNEY   TOKYO

W.B. SAUNDERS COMPANY
A Division of Elsevier Inc.

1600 John F. Kennedy Boulevard, Suite 1800 • Philadelphia, Pennsylvania 19103-2899

http://www.theclinics.com

ANESTHESIOLOGY CLINICS

March 2007

Editor: Rachel Glover

Volume 25, Number 1
ISSN 1932-2275
ISBN-13: 978-1-4160-4278-5
ISBN-10: 1-4160-4278-4

The ideas and opinions expressed in *Anesthesiology Clinics* do not necessarily reflect those of the Publisher. The Publisher does not assume any responsibility for any injury and/or damage to persons or property arising out of or related to any use of the material contained in this periodical. The reader is advised to check the appropriate medical literature and the product information currently provided by the manufacturer of each drug to be administered to verify the dosage, the method and duration of administration, or contraindications. It is the responsibility of the treating physician or other health care professional, relying on independent experience and knowledge of the patient, to determine drug dosages and the best treatment for the patient. Mention of any product in this issue should not be construed as endorsement by the contributors, editors, or the Publisher of the product or manufacturers' claims.

Anesthesiology Clinics (ISSN 1932-2275) is published quarterly by Elsevier Inc., 360 Park Avenue South, New York, NY 10010-1710. Months of issue are March, June, September, and December. Business and Editorial Offices: 1600 John F. Kennedy Blvd., Suite 1800, Philadelphia, PA 19103-2899. Customer Service Office: 6277 Sea Harbor Drive, Orlando, FL 32887-4800. Periodicals postage paid at New York, NY and additional mailing offices. Subscription prices are $101.00 per year (US student/resident), $202.00 per year (US individuals), $246.00 per year (Canadian individuals), $302.00 per year (US institutions), $366.00 per year (Canadian institutions), $134.00 per year (Canadian and foreign student/resident), $263.00 per year (foreign individuals), and $366.00 per year (foreign institutions). To receive student and resident rate, orders must be accompanied by name of affiliated institution, date of term, and the *signature* of program/residency coordinator on institutions letterhead. Orders will be billed at individual rate until proof of status is received. Foreign air speed delivery is included in all *Clinics'* subscription prices. All prices are subject to change without notice. POSTMASTER: Send address changes to *Anesthesiology Clinics*, Elsevier Periodicals Customer Service, 6277 Sea Harbor Drive, Orlando, FL 32887-4800. **Customer Service: 1-800-654-2452** (US). From outside of the US, call **1-407-345-4000**. E-mail: hhspcs@wbsaunders.com.

Anesthesiology Clinics, is also published in Spanish by McGraw-Hill Inter-americana Editores S. A., P.O. Box 5-237, 06500 Mexico D. F., Mexico.

Anesthesiology Clinics, is covered in *Index Medicus, Current Contents/Clinical Medicine, Excerpta Medica, ISI/BIOMED*, and *Chemical Abstracts*.

Printed in the United States of America.

CONSULTING EDITOR

LEE A. FLEISHER, MD, Robert D. Dripps Professor and Chair, Department of Anesthesiology and Critical Care, The University of Pennsylvania School of Medicine, Philadelphia, Pennsylvania

GUEST EDITORS

MICHA Y. SHAMIR, MD, Instructor, Department of Anesthesiology and Critical Care Medicine, Hadassah-Hebrew University Medical Center, Hadassah-Hebrew University Medical School, Jerusalem, Israel

YORAM G. WEISS, MD, Senior Lecturer, Department of Anesthesiology and Critical Care Medicine, Hadassah-Hebrew University Medical Center, Hadassah-Hebrew University Medical School, Jerusalem, Israel; Department of Anesthesiology and Critical Care, University of Pennsylvania School of Medicine, Philadelphia, PA

CONTRIBUTORS

KARIM ABOUELENIN, MD, Assistant Professor of Clinical Anesthesiology, Miller School of Medicine at the University of Miami, Miami, Florida

BRUCE C. BAKER, CAPT, MC, USN, Naval Hospital, Camp Pendleton, California

DAVID J. BAKER, DM, FRCA, Consultant Anesthesiologist, Department of Anesthesiology and SAMU de Paris, Hôpital Nècker–Enfants Malades, Paris, France

DIMITRY BARANOV, MD, Assistant Professor, Anesthesiology and Critical Care, Hospital of University of Pennsylvania, Philadelphia, Pennsylvania

HAIM BERKENSTADT, MD, Director of Neuroanesthesia, Department of Anesthesiology and Intensive Care, Sheba Medical Center, Tel Hashomer; and Deputy Director, The Israel Center for Medical Simulation, Sheba Medical Center, Tel Hashomer, Tel Aviv University, Sackler School of Medicine, Tel Aviv, Israel

GEORGE J. BRAND, LT, NC, USN, 1st Medical Battalion, Camp Pendleton, California

STEPHEN J. BRETT, MD, FRCA, Consultant in Intensive Care Medicine, Department of Anaesthesia and Intensive Care, Hammersmith Hospital, London, United Kingdom

CHESTER (TRIP) BUCKENMAIER, LTC, MC, USA, Walter Reed Army Medical Center, Washington, District of Columbia

PIERRE CARLI, MD, PhD, Professor of Anesthesiology Director, Department of Anesthesiology and SAMU de Paris, Hôpital Nècker–Enfants Malades, Paris, France

MAURIZIO CEREDA, MD, Clinical Assistant Professor, Department of Anesthesiology and Critical Care, University of Pennsylvania, Philadelphia, Pennsylvania; Staff Anesthesiologist, Philadelphia VA Medical Center, Philadelphia, Pennsylvania

MICHAEL E. COMPEGGIE, LCDR MC, USN, Naval Hospital, Camp LeJeune, North Carolina

JAMES G. CUSHMAN, MD, Associate Professor of Surgery, Department of Surgery, University of Maryland, R. Adams Cowley Shock Trauma Center, Baltimore, Maryland

ROSARIO CUSIMANO, MD, Attending Physician, Dipartimento Emergenza Accettazione, ASO CTO-CRF-Maria Adelaide, Torino, Italy

DANIELA DECAROLI, MD, Attending Physcician, Dipartimento Emergenza Accettazione, ASO CTO-CRF-Maria Adelaide, Torino, Italy

CLIFFORD S. DEUTSCHMAN, MD, Professor, Department of Anesthesiology and Critical Care, University of Pennsylvania, Philadelphia, Pennsylvania

JACQUES DURANTEAU, MD, PhD, Professor, Department of Critical Care and Anesthesiology, University Paris XI, Bicêtre Hospital, Paris, France

RICHARD P. DUTTON, MD, MBA, Associate Professor of Anesthesiology, University of Maryland School of Medicine; Director, Division of Trauma Anesthesiology, R Adams Cowley Shock Trauma Center, University of Maryland Medical System, Baltimore, Maryland

URIEL ELCHALAL, MD, Senior Lecturer in Obstetrics and Gynecology, Department of Obstetrics and Gynecology, Hadassah Hebrew University Medical Center, Ein Karem, Jerusalem, Israel

DAVID EREZ, EMT-P, MSc, Programs Director, The Israel Center for Medical Simulation, Sheba Medical Center, Tel Hashomer, Tel Aviv University, Sackler School of Medicine, Tel Aviv, Israel

MAJOR JEFF GARNER, MB ChB, MRCS(Ed), RAMC, Specialist Registrar in General Surgery, Northern General Hospital, Sheffield, United Kingdom

YEHUDA GINOSAR, BSc, MBBS, Lecturer in Anesthesiology, Department of Anesthesiology and Critical Care Medicine, Hadassah Hebrew University Medical Center, Ein Karem, Jerusalem, Israel

YAACOV GOZAL, MD, Associate Professor of Anesthesiology; Director, Operating Rooms and PACU, Department of Anesthesiology & CCM, Hadassah Hebrew University School of Medicine, Hadassah Medical Organization, Jerusalem, Israel

CESARE GREGORETTI, MD, Chief, Dipartimento Emergenza Accettazione, ASO CTO-CRF-Maria Adelaide, Torino, Italy

MICHAEL C. LEWIS, MD, Associate Professor of Clinical Anesthesiology, Miller School of Medicine at the University of Miami, Miami, Florida

RICHARD R. McNEER, MD, PhD, Assistant Professor, Department of Anesthesiology Perioperative Medicine and Pain Management, Ryder Trauma Center, Miller School of Medicine, University of Miami, Miami, Florida

YUVAL MEROZ, MD, Instructor in Anesthesiology, Department of Anesthesiology and Critical Care Medicine, Hadassah Hebrew University Medical Center, Ein Karem, Jerusalem, Israel

ANTONIO MILETTO, MD, Chief, Dipartimento Emergenza Accettazione, ASO CTO-CRF-Maria Adelaide, Torino, Italy

ALICE MISTRETTA, MD, Fellow, Università di Torino, Dipartimento di Anestesiologia e Rianimazione, Ospedale S. Giovanni Battista-Molinette Torino, Torino, Italy

PAUL D. MONGAN, COL, MC, USA, Department of Anesthesiology, The Uniformed Services University, Walter Reed Army Medical Center, Washington, District of Columbia

YARON MUNZ, MD, Senior Surgeon, Department of Surgery and Transplantation, Sheba Medical Center, Tel Hashomer; and Director of Surgical Simulation Programs, The Israel Center for Medical Simulation, Sheba Medical Center, Tel Hashomer, Tel Aviv University, Sackler School of Medicine, Tel Aviv, Israel

NALAN NARINE, CDR, MC, USN, Naval Hospital, Camp Pendleton, California

PATRICK NELIGAN, MA, MD, Assistant Professor, Anesthesiology and Critical Care, Hospital of University of Pennsylvania, Philadelphia, Pennsylvania

MIGUEL PANIAGUA, MD, Assistant Professor of Medicine, Division of Gerontology & Geriatric Medicine and Miami VA GRECC, Miller School of Medicine at the University of Miami, Miami, Florida

EDGAR J. PIERRE, MD, Assistant Professor, Department of Anesthesiology Perioperative Medicine and Pain Management, Ryder Trauma Center, Miller School of Medicine, University of Miami, Miami, Florida

V. MARCO RANIERI, MD, Professor, Università di Torino, Dipartimento di Anestesiologia e Rianimazione, Ospedale S. Giovanni Battista-Molinette Torino, Torino, Italy

J. DAVID ROCCAFORTE, MD, Assistant Professor, Department of Anesthesiology, New York University, New York; Co-Director SICU, Department of Anesthesia, Bellevue Hospital, New York, New York

ROLF ROSSAINT, MD, PhD, Professor and Head, Department of Anesthesiology, Aachen University, Aachen, Germany

MICHA Y. SHAMIR, MD, Instructor, Department of Anesthesiology and Critical Care Medicine, Hadassah-Hebrew University Medical Center, Hadassah-Hebrew University Medical School, Jerusalem, Israel

DANIEL SIMON, MD, Director of Trauma Unit, Sheba Medical Center, Tel Hashomer, Tel Aviv University, Sackler School of Medicine, Tel Aviv, Israel

DONAT R. SPAHN, MD, FRCA, Professor, Department of Anaesthesiology, University Hospital Lausanne, Lausanne, Switzerland

PHILIP F. STAHEL, MD, Professor, Department of Orthopedic Surgery, Denver Health Medical Center, University of Colorado School of Medicine, Denver, Colorado

DANIEL TALMOR, MD, MPH, Director of Trauma Anesthesia and Critical Care, Department of Anesthesia and Critical Care, Beth Israel Deaconess Medical Center; Assistant Professor, Harvard Medical School, Boston, Massachusetts

CAROLINE TELION, MD, Consultant Anesthesiologist, Department of Anesthesiology and SAMU de Paris, Hôpital Nècker–Enfants Malades, Paris, France

YORAM G. WEISS, MD, Senior Lecturer, Department of Anesthesiology and Critical Care Medicine, Hadassah-Hebrew University Medical Center, Hadassah-Hebrew University Medical School, Jerusalem, Israel; Department of Anesthesiology and Critical Care, University of Pennsylvania School of Medicine, Philadelphia, PA

AMITAI ZIV, MD, Director, The Israel Center for Medical Simulation, Sheba Medical Center, Tel Hashomer; and Deputy Director for Patient Safety and Medical Education, Sheba Medical Center, Tel Hashomer, Tel Aviv University, Sackler School of Medicine, Tel Aviv, Israel

CONTENTS

> Penetrating face and neck trauma is usually obvious, but blunt trauma mandates high index of suspicion to recognize its existence. Comprehensive understanding of the injury is mandatory to plan the best timing and method to secure the airway.

> Patients admitted to the ICU after severe trauma require frequent procedures in the operating room, particularly in cases where a damage control strategy is used. The ventilatory management of these patients in the operating room can be particularly challenging. These patients often have severely impaired respiratory mechanics because of acute lung injury and abdominal compartment syndrome. Consequently, the pressure and flow generation capabilities of standard anesthesia ventilators may be inadequate to support ventilation and gas exchange. This article presents the problems that may be encountered in patients who have severe abdominal and lung injuries, and the current management concepts used in caring for these patients in the critical care setting, to provide guidelines for the anesthetist faced with these patients in the operating room.

professionals. The diverse range of medical simulation modalities enables trainees to acquire and practice an array of tasks and skills. SBME offers the field of trauma training multiple opportunities to enhance the effectiveness of the education provided in this challenging domain. In this article, the authors describe the possible roles of simulated patients, skills trainers, computerized patient simulators, and web-based teaching in trauma training, and describe some practical aspects of using simulation for trauma training.

Modern society is characterized as having an ever enlarging population of older adults. There are more elderly patients, and the average age of this group is increasing. The anesthetic management of surgery for the elderly trauma victim is more complicated than in younger adults. Evaluation of the physiologic status of the geriatric patient should take into account the variability of the changes associated with advancing age. Care of the injured elderly patient requires thorough preoperative assessment and planning and the involvement of a multidisciplinary clinical team knowledgeable about and interested in the management of the elderly surgical patient.

Obese persons are more likely to be involved in vehicle accidents, probably because of the presence of sleep apnea. They are more likely to suffer chest, pelvis, and extremity fractures. Mildly overweight persons are less prone to intra-abdominal injury because of the protective effect of the abdominal fat, known as the cushion effect. Obese trauma patients are far more likely to develop in-hospital complications, especially pulmonary, renal, and thromboembolic complications. The BMI is an independent risk factor for morbidity and mortality after trauma. Because only limited data exist about the right clinical approach to obese trauma patients, it is necessary to rely on general knowledge about treating obese patients in the ICU. More research is needed to improve the treatment of obese trauma patients.

Medical and surgical treatment of the trauma patient has evolved in the last decade. Treatment of pain from multiple fractures or injured organs and surgical anesthesia with regional anesthesia techniques have been used to reduce post-traumatic stress disorder and reduce the adverse effects of general anesthesia. Neuraxial blocks and peripheral nerve block techniques should be practiced by trained emergency and operatory room staff. This article reviews recent publications related to the role of regional anesthesia in trauma patients in the prehospital, emergency, and operatory room settings. It also describes indications, limitations, and practical aspects of regional anesthesia.

The principles enshrined in existing trauma resuscitation protocols for treating nonpregnant trauma victims should also be applied to the pregnant patient. In addition, left tilt of the pregnant patient (or the back board) and supplement oxygen are mandatory. The patient should be treated by a multidisciplinary team, preferably in a trauma center. Early intubation is recommended, but should be performed, where possible, by an experienced physician. The physician should be aware of the different physiologic and laboratory values in normal pregnancy. Fetal monitoring is important to assess both fetal and maternal welfare. Imaging examinations, where indicated, should not be delayed. Even minor maternal trauma, especially if caused by interpersonal violence, might cause fetal loss.

Expeditionary maneuver warfare and the asymmetric battlefield have forced changes in the traditional methods with which we deliver anesthesia and surgery to the wounded. Although in many ways similar to how we have operated on the wounded for the past half century, new advances in diagnostic and therapeutic modalities and doctrinal shifts have changed the face of the battlefield hospital. In this article, the authors discuss these changes in regard to anesthetic care for surgical and pain management for wounded airmen, sailors, soldiers, and marines.

Explosive devices cause injury by four mechanisms, of which primary blast injury is the least familiar to most non-military clinicians. The pathophysiology of the various mechanisms of injury is described, and the implications for translating a knowledge of mechanism of injury to clinical management is discussed.

FORTHCOMING ISSUES

RECENT ISSUES

ANESTHESIOLOGY
CLINICS

Anesthesiology Clin
25 (2007) xiii–xiv

Foreword

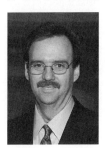

Lee A. Fleisher, MD
Consulting Editor

Trauma is a multifaceted issue, with victims ranging widely in age and usually with unknown medical histories. The nature of trauma itself is to be unpredictable, with causes ranging from automobile accidents, to violent crime, to terrorism, with the number and severity of injuries as yet another variable. It is therefore very appropriate to focus an issue of *Anesthesiology Clinics* on this constantly evolving area. It is an unfortunate truth that, in a world of political turmoil, war, and terrorism, trauma can increasingly be considered a global pandemic. We are, therefore, fortunate to have two distinguished authors from the Hadassah Medical Center in Jerusalem to edit this issue. Drs. Yoram Weiss and Micha Shamir have developed an issue of *Clinics* with viewpoints from multiple international perspectives.

Dr. Weiss is a Senior Lecturer in Anesthesiology in the Department of Anesthesiology & Critical Care Medicine at Hadassah, Hebrew University, Jerusalem and an Adjunct Assistant Professor of Anesthesia at the University of Pennsylvania, Philadelphia, Pennsylvania. Since 2002, Dr. Weiss has been an instructor in advanced trauma life support courses, as well as a member of the Committee on the Management of the Severe Head Injury Patient for the Israeli National Council for Surgery Anesthetics and Intensive Care in the Ministry of Health. He has lectured on topics such as Acute Respiratory Distress Syndrome (ARDS) and blast injury and has authored papers dealing with the effects of terrorism, such as "Blast lung injury from an explosion on a civilian bus" [1] and "Multiple casualty terror events: the anesthesiologist's perspective" in *Anesthesia and Analgesia*. He also has written on tension pneumoperitoneum after blast injury for the *Journal of*

Trauma, and was a coauthor of a chapter on acute lung injuries among survivors from suicide bomb attacks.

Micha Y. Shamir, M.D., is an Instructor in Anesthesiology in the Department of Anesthesiology & Critical Care Medicine at Hadassah, Hebrew University, Jerusalem. He has written extensively about the anesthesiologist's perspective on trauma patients in papers such as "Multiple casualty terror events: the anesthesiologist's perspective" in *Anesthesia and Analgesia* and "The Israeli experience:conventional terrorism and critical care" in *Critical Care* as well as papers on suicide bombings. He has also lectured on such subjects as hemorrhagic shock, airway management in trauma, and injury by explosive device.

These two editors have put together an outstanding issue, which can be used to keep those in our specialty informed of the latest developments in treatment of the trauma patient.

Lee A. Fleisher, MD
Department of Anesthesiology and Critical Care
The University of Pennsylvania School of Medicine
3400 Spruce Street, Dulles 600
Philadelphia, PA 19104, USA

E-mail address: fleishel@uphs.upenn.edu

Reference

[1] Pizov R, Oppenheim-Eden A, Matot I, et al. Blast lung injury from an explosion on a civilian bus. Chest 1999;115(1):165–72.

ELSEVIER
SAUNDERS

Anesthesiology Clin
25 (2007) xv–xvii

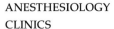

ANESTHESIOLOGY
CLINICS

Preface

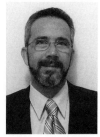 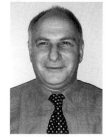

Micha Y. Shamir, MD   Yoram G. Weiss, MD
Guest Editors

Trauma is one of the most common causes of death, especially in young people. The high incidence of trauma explains why anesthesiologists are treating increasing numbers of trauma victims. Participation of anesthesiologists in the resuscitation of trauma victims is important because they are trained to provide advanced airway management, shock resuscitation, and invasive monitoring.

Better motor vehicle safety, combined with better organized and trained prehospital services have improved the survival of severely injured patients admitted to medical centers. This is demonstrated by the constant increase in the "survival to hospital" of patients with very high Injury Severity Scores (ISS). Some of these patients will survive and resume normal lives. These impressive successes are attributed to multidisciplinary team efforts in which novel approaches were introduced by the various disciplines. One of the most important is the use of invasive angiographic procedures to place stents and selectively embolize bleeding blood vessels. These procedures have replaced extremely complicated vascular surgeries. Another major novel approach is damage control procedures aiming to reduce multisystem organ failure and death by firstly stabilizing devastating abdominal injuries.

Recent demographic trends complicated the care of trauma victims as they are associated with an older trauma population. This change is a reflection of the constant increase in many countries in mean life expectancy from 65 to almost 80 over the last 20 years. The elderly trauma patient presents a challenge because of significant underlying chronic disorders coupled with

1932-2275/07/$ - see front matter © 2007 Elsevier Inc. All rights reserved.
doi:10.1016/j.anclin.2007.01.001   *anesthesiology.theclinics.com*

a multidrug regimen. Finally, the significant increase in prevalence of morbid obesity disorders in the western population demands special attention.

The trauma issue of *Anesthesiology Clinics of North America* is organized into three sectors: current trauma practices, special populations, and terrorism. The contributors were selected to present both American and European trauma experiences and approaches.

The first section of this issue discusses "problem-oriented" issues such as securing the injured airway, initiation of intensive care unit treatment in the operating room, aggressive homeostatic efforts, and management of hemorrhage and shock. A relatively new concept presented is conservative treatment to hemodynamic instability and the transition from aggressive resuscitative regimens to hypotensive resuscitation. Similarly, bleeding control is now part of the invasive radiologist's practice. Lastly, pharmacologic treatments for bleeding problems have been introduced including fibrinogen concentrates and recombinant factor VIIa. The latter was introduced within the last 4 years as an "off-label indication" for the treatment of exsanguinations. Currently, no human level 1 or 2 scientific support exists to justify its use in trauma. The first double-blind, randomized trauma study did not find a decrease in mortality rate [1]. Recently, the US Food and Drug Administration raised serious doubts about the safety of its use in trauma patients [2]. Currently, a major double-blind study is being conducted in the United States, and its results are eagerly awaited.

The second section discusses the treatment of special high-risk populations, including obese, pregnant, and elderly trauma victims. Treating these populations mandates aggressive supportive measures to improve outcome. To do so, creative anesthetic regimens, such as the use of regional anesthesia in trauma, have been introduced.

The last section addresses the consequences of terrorism. Unfortunately, it is generally accepted today that terror can hit anywhere at anytime. These chapters portray the experience gained in dealing with the aftermath of terror. We chose to present the experience gathered after major terror events in New York, London, and Paris and by the US Army. Finally, chemical and biologic warfare are becoming an increasing menace to our societies. However, a thorough review of these issues is beyond the scope of this issue. Hence, we included a review of the only nonconventional chemical, organophosphate, used in a Japanese terror incident.

Micha Y. Shamir, MD
Yoram G. Weiss, MD
Department of Anesthesiology and Critical Care Medicine
Hadassah – Hebrew University Medical Center
Hadassah – Hebrew University Medical School
P.O. Box 12000, Jerusalem 91120, Israel

E-mail address: shamir61@gmail.com

References

[1] Boffard KD, Riou B, Warren B, et al. Recombinant factor VIIa as adjunctive therapy for bleeding control in severely injured trauma patients: two parallel randomized, placebo-controlled, double-blind clinical trials. J Trauma 2005;59:8–18.

[2] O'Connell KA, Wood JJ, Wise RP, et al. Thromboemlolic adverse events after use of recombinant human coagulation factor VIIa. JAMA 2006;295:293–8.

ANESTHESIOLOGY
CLINICS

Anesthesiology Clin
25 (2007) 1–11

Early Management of the Traumatized Airway

Edgar J. Pierre, MD[a,*],
Richard R. McNeer, MD, PhD[a],
Micha Y. Shamir, MD[a,b]

[a]Department of Anesthesiology Perioperative Medicine and Pain Management,
Ryder Trauma Center, Miller School of Medicine, University of Miami,
Miami, FL 33136, USA
[b]Department of Anesthesiology and Critical Care Medicine, Hadassah – Hebrew University
Hospital, Jerusalem, Israel

The primary survey ("ABC" algorithm) in a trauma victim involves rapid evaluation and stabilization of vital functions that are crucial to survival. As a part of the "A" (airway) assessment it is necessary to determine whether there is an immediate need to artificially secure the airway.

Trauma to the face and neck might cause life-threatening injuries to the upper airway, vascular structures, cervical spine, and aerodigestive tract. The goal of airway intervention is to relieve or prevent airway obstruction and to secure the unprotected airway from aspiration. This goal can be difficult to achieve in the traumatized airway because of the frequent presence of blood, secretions, tissue edema, and debris (such as avulsed teeth and tissue) that can interfere with the identification of the airway anatomy, which may already be distorted. In addition, the stomach is assumed to be full and the cervical spine unstable, which increases difficulty when managing the airway. As a consequence, managing the traumatized airway can prove to be the ultimate test of a physician's technical skills, which includes familiarity with available equipment and airway management strategies and the ability to improvise under stressful and often fast-changing circumstances.

Once the airway is secured, a meticulous diagnostic workup is to be started to verify the exact location of injury and to choose the appropriate surgical intervention. This may include fiberoptic examination of the

* Corresponding author. Division of Trauma and Critical Care Medicine, Department of Anesthesiology, University of Miami, Ryder Trauma Center, 1800 NW 10 Ave., Miami, FL 33136.

E-mail address: pierre@miami.edu (E.J. Pierre).

0889-8537/07/$ - see front matter © 2007 Elsevier Inc. All rights reserved.
doi:10.1016/j.anclin.2006.11.001 *anesthesiology.theclinics.com*

pharynx, larynx, trachea, and esophagus. Other modalities can include chest and neck radiographs, computed tomography, angiography, and contrast swallow fluoroscopy. This workup is beyond the scoop of this review.

With these general points in mind, the remainder of this chapter will discuss the unique challenges and solutions that present in patients with maxillofacial trauma and neck injury (laryngotracheal injury and neck hematoma).

Neck injuries

The neck contains multiple vital structures including the main airway, cervical spinal cord/nerves, and blood vessels. Injury to the neck, therefore, carries high rate of mortality and morbidity. Mortality is as high as 40% for laryngotracheal injury associated with blunt trauma and 20% for those associated with penetrating trauma [1,2].

Laryngotracheal trauma

Historically, most laryngotracheal injuries were the result of blunt trauma to the cervical region. Lately it seems that that there is a shift in the mechanism toward penetrating injuries [3]. Inside the blunt trauma group, there is also a shift toward more victims of motorcycle crashes instead of car accidents [2]. This shift might be the result of increased crime rate. Concomitantly, it might reflect improved automobile safety, lower speed limits, and mandatory use of safety belts [3]. Obstructive injury to the airway is the second most common cause of death associated with trauma to the head and neck [4]. Mild to moderate trauma may cause tissue edema, hematoma, or mucosal tears. Severe injuries can result in disruption of the airway, neurovascular bundle, and visceral rupture [5]. Fortunately, injuries to the cervical aerodigestive tract are uncommon, ranging from 1.2% in blunt trauma to 10.2% in penetrating injuries to the neck [6]. The most important injuries in the neck include: (1) partial or total disruption of tracheal continuity, (2) fractures of larynx/cricoid obstructing the airway, (3) major arterial/venous bleeding leading to hemorrhagic shock or hematoma formation that compresses or obstructs the airway, (4) cervical spine injury causing apnea or neurogenic shock or perforation of the esophagus.

Penetrating neck trauma can be caused by gunshot, knife, or other foreign bodies. These injuries are usually described according to the entrance site as one of three zones of the neck (Fig. 1). An alternative classification describes the neck as anterolateral or posterior portions divided by the sternocleidomastoid muscle. This classification stems from the observation that injury to the anterolateral part of the neck is more dangerous because of the proximity to the trachea, larynx, and cervical vessels [7].

Blunt trauma to the neck that produces laryngotracheal injury may be caused by three mechanisms: (1) direct, such as collision with a vehicular

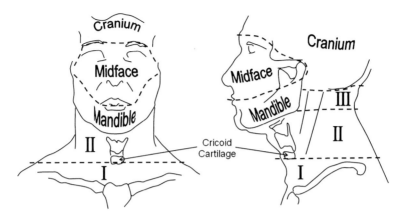

Fig. 1. Classification of facial and neck zones of injury. The zones of the face are described as either midfacial or mandibular. Injuries in both zones can lead to airway obstruction and difficult ventilation. Visualization during direct laryngoscopy may be aided in the presence of mandibular fractures. The neck is divided in to three zones. Zone I extends from the clavicles to the cricoid cartilage, and injury in this zone carries high mortality rate. In addition to neck organs it contains upper thoracic lung and blood vessels. Zone II lies between the cricoid and the mandibular angle. It contains major cervical arteries and veins as well as extrathoracic air and food tracts. It is the most frequently injured area, and the mortality rate is lower because of easy surgical access. Zone III comprises the area between the base of skull and the angle of the mandible. This area is also difficult to approach surgically [16].

dashboard, a human assault, sports injury, fall from height, and hanging; (2) deceleration injury, such as car accidents and fall from height that can produce shearing injuries to fixed organs such as the cricoid cartilage or tracheal carina; and (3) increased pressure, such as sudden antero-posterior chest compression against a closed glottis that can cause abrupt increases in intrathoracic pressure, resulting in linear rupture of the posterior membranous trachea [1,8].

In contrast to blunt neck injuries, penetrating injuries usually are obvious. As a result, physician attention may be distracted from assessment of other coexisting life-threatening injuries such as head or chest trauma [9]. Blunt neck trauma can be associated with other more impressive injuries in 50% or more of cases. Hence, co-existing injuries might mask potentially lethal neck injury from blunt trauma (eg, spine and maxillofacial fractures, chest trauma, and closed head injuries) [1]. Diagnosis of blunt neck trauma depends on a high index of suspicion [4].

Clinical examination remains the most reliable sign of laryngotracheal injury. The only hard diagnostic sign to airway trauma is air leaking through the neck wound. Other signs and symptoms include subcutaneous emphysema, dyspnea, hemoptysis, dysphonia (from hoarseness to aphonia), stridor, cough, hemoptysis, and crepitance upon palpation [2,8–10]. Soft tissue swelling is responsible for the sensation of choking, dyspnea, dysphagia, hoarseness, and stridor experienced by these patients [5]. Transcervical gunshot wounds evidenced radiographically or by the existence of entrance and contralateral exit wounds carry high risk for major vascular or visceral damage [10]. Crepitus on palpation of the cricoid/tracheal cartilages is of the utmost importance in diagnostic airway injury.

The quality of the victim's voice (ie, hoarseness) is important. A hoarse voice indicates major airway injury until proven otherwise [11]. This finding should never be overlooked unless the patient is alert and can verify the existence of hoarseness before the injury. Information from prehospital providers documenting the development of hoarseness should immediately alert the anesthesiologist to the presence of an airway injury.

Patients with blunt laryngotracheal injury require emergency airway in almost 79% of cases, whereas those with penetrating require it in 46% of cases. The requirement for emergency airway is a significant predictor of mortality [3]. The most urgent priority in penetrating and blunt neck trauma is securing the airway. The end result should be an endotracheal tube with an inflated sealing cuff positioned entirely distal to a laryngotracheal perforation. Nevertheless, intubation of the trachea might be extremely difficult because pharyngeal or neck hematoma might obscure the vocal cords or distort the anatomy. Blind advancement of the endotracheal tube in the trachea can be dangerous because it might follow/cause a false route or complete a transected airway [8,12]. The obvious conclusion is to avoid tracheal intubation at the scene or emergency department (as long as the patient is stable). The more common neck injuries (stab wounds and lowvelocity gunshots) usually do not mandate prehospital or emergency department intubation. Intubation should be performed in the operating room by the most experienced available anesthesia provider, with the proper equipment and availability to perform surgical interventions. On the contrary, high-velocity gun shot bullets and severe blunt neck injuries often mandate urgent airway control at the scene [8].

The laryngeal mask airway, rapid sequence orotracheal intubation, and esophageal obturator are contraindicated in patients suspected to have laryngotracheal discontinuation. If rapid sequence orotracheal intubation is necessary, concomitant preparation for fiberoptic confirmation of the proper tube position is mandatory as well as continuing preparations for the establishment of a surgical airway (cricothyroidotomy) establishment. Emergency tracheotomy is not considered an appropriate method to establish emergency for the reasons described above.

The unstable patient with a slash wound to the throat can be intubated through the incision as a life-saving act [12]. For prehospital personnel, cricothyroidotomy is practically the only appropriate alternative if artificial airway establishment cannot be delayed until arrival at the hospital.

Blind intubation should not be used in patients with potential laryngotracheal injury because of the risk of complete airway obstruction. Either routine intubation or a tracheostomy can secure the airway. A tracheostomy provides space with which to examine the site of injury both at the site and from above with direct laryngoscopy. Endotracheal intubation might render further examination of the injury difficult and might aggravate an existing injury. However, there is controversy regarding the best method of gaining a secure airway [3,13]. In the past, cricothyroidotomy or tracheotomy was the procedure of choice even in the hospital [1]. Recent literature allows for orotracheal intubation, providing it is done under direct vision of a broncho-scope, thus ensuring that the entire path of the tube is intraluminar. Using a bronchoscope is also helpful in placing the entirety of the sealing cuff distal to the perforation in the trachea [6,7]. In a series of 71 patients with laryngeal tracheal trauma, 39 (54.9%) required an emergency airway. Forty-eight per-cent of patients underwent initial orotracheal intubation, whereas tracheos-tomy and cricothyroidotomy were performed in 4% each. Patients with blunt laryngeal tracheal trauma required an emergency airway in 78.9% of cases, whereas those with penetrating injuries required one in 46.2% of cases. Intubation was successful in 14 of the 15 patients in the blunt trauma group and 20 of the 24 patients in the penetrating trauma group [2,3,13,14].

Laryngeal tracheal trauma remains a rare and life-threatening set of injuries with serious complications. To reduce the risk of adverse outcomes in this patient population, a team approach (anesthesiologist, surgeons, and support personnel) should be well educated in the management of upper air-way injuries.

Neck hematoma

Neck hematoma could be the result of penetrating or blunt trauma. Many patients suffering neck hematoma are elderly people under chronic anticoag-ulant therapy who sustained a relative minor injury [5]. Signs of vascular in-juries are hematoma (Fig. 2), hypotension, and persistent bleeding [5]. The hematoma can be limited without jeopardizing the airway; however, bleeding and edema may gradually or rapidly enlarge. In this case, a critical point may abruptly be reached in which the airway will be obstructed, and the patient's condition will deteriorate [5]. It is reasonable to postpone tracheal intubation until arrival at the hospital because of the inability to predict the clinical course and the possibility of a difficult tracheal intubation (bulging hematoma and soft tissue swelling). Nevertheless, close monitoring of the patient and evalu-ation of the size of the hematoma is crucial. Preventive intubation should be done if the hematoma enlarges or if the patient shows progressive signs of airway compromise. A low threshold for intubation is advocated if the evac-uation time is long or if the health provider's skills are limited (less experience mandates intubation before anatomy significantly distorts). In the field, emer-gency department, and operating room, "difficult intubation" should be antic-ipated, and the technique should be planned accordingly.

Facial and pharyngeal trauma

Traumatic injury to the face and upper airway poses particular difficulties (see Fig. 1). Failure to identify an injury to the face or neck can lead to acute

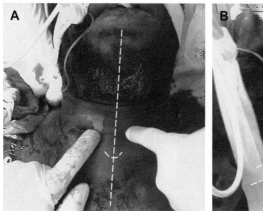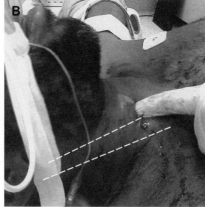

Fig. 2. Penetrating trauma to the neck. The surgeon's finger is present (inserted) in the wound (*A* and *B*). Note that the anesthesiologist's finger marks the site of the midline of the cricoid cartilage (*A*). The location of the wound is at the border of zones I and II (*A*) and anterior to the sternocleidomastoid muscle outlined by the two dashed lines (*B*). The larynx and trachea are deviated from midline (single dashed line) secondary to a rapidly expanding hematoma on the side of injury (*A*). The "u"-shaped dashed line represents the suprasternal notch (*A*). The patient was in shock, and airway management involved performing a fiber optic rapid sequence intubation.

airway obstruction secondary to swelling and hematoma. Significant injury to the upper airway is uncommon, with a reported incidence of 0.03% to 2.8% of all trauma patients. The frequency is 1 case per 30,000 emergency department evaluations [1]. Most upper airway injuries are secondary to direct blunt or penetrating trauma (knife or gunshot) or severe flexion–extension injuries. The patient with blunt or penetrating injury to the midface, mandible, or oral cavity is at risk for brain damage or death from upper airway obstruction [15].

Fragmentation of bone and teeth and disruption of adjacent soft tissues characterize severe injuries of the mandible (Fig. 3). Tears of the floor of the mouth can extend to the pharynx, tonsil, submaxillary triangle, and hyoid bone.

Midface fractures or LeFort fractures of the maxilla, present difficult clinical problems. Motion of the maxilla independent of the remainder of the face indicates a LeFort I fracture. In addition, the LeFort II fracture can extend through the orbital rim, medial orbital wall, ethmoid sinuses, and nose. Injury of the ethmoid sinus roof or cribiform plate may result in cerebrospinal fluid rhinorrhea, meningitis, or temporary or permanent loss of smell. LeFort III fracture is a transverse fracture above the malar bone and through the orbits. It is characterized by complete separation of the maxilla from the craniofacial skeleton, epistaxis, and a flat dish-face deformity [11]. Evaluation of midface fractures is confirmed with computed tomography scans in the axial and coronal planes. In certain situations, a three-dimensional reconstruction is useful [5].

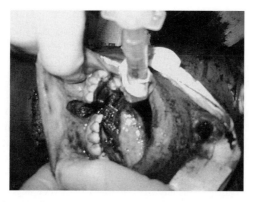

Fig. 3. Traumatic fracture of the mandible after a gunshot wound to the mandible. Avulsed teeth, presence of blood and distorted anatomy can make airway management difficult. Rapid sequence intubation with a suction catheter in the mouth was performed, and a grade I laryngoscopy was appreciated.

Penetrating trauma to the face can be described by a number of facial zone divisions. The simplest one divides the face into midface and mandibular zones (see Fig. 1). Practically all stab wounds and most gunshot wounds (71%) are to the midface zone [14].

Injury to the cervical spine co-exists in 0 to 4% of the patients suffering facial trauma [16]. Hyperextension of the head during laryngoscopy introduces the risk of spinal cord transection in the presence of an unstable vertebral fracture and is a very significant coexisting injury vis a vis airway management. Life-threatening hypovolemia is uncommon as a result of isolated facial trauma occurring only in 1% to 4% of the patients [17]. Tears in the dura occur in 25% of all Le Fort II and III fractures, along with leakage of cerebrospinal fluid [11]. Other injuries of an immediate concern regarding the airway are head and vascular injuries [14].

Most facial injuries are obvious and can be recognized by hemorrhage, edema, erythema, and facial distortion. In a minority of cases, mainly isolated facial blunt trauma, edema, and erythema might not appear in the very early stages. In this case, crepitus on palpation, hoarse voice, drooling, and refusal to obtain the supine posture should alert for facial injury or airway injury.

Because of its urgency, assessment of the airway should be almost entirely clinical. Important findings to note include anxiety, stridor, ability to phonate, and movement of air through the mouth and nares, tracheal deviation, the use of accessory muscles of respiration, and movement of the diaphragm.

Intra-oral hemorrhage, pharyngeal erythema, and change in voice are all indications for early intubation. Mandibular injuries are more prone for the need of early intubation. Bilateral mandibular fractures and pharyngeal hemorrhage may lead to upper airway obstruction, particularly in a supine patient. Therefore, a patient found in the sitting or prone position because of airway compromise is best left in that position until the moment of anesthetic induction and intubation [11].

Airway management should begin with assessment of the urgency of which intubation should be done. Usually facial injuries will posses a difficult intubation issue and not impossible intubation [18]. An oral or nasopharyngeal airway may be required to temporarily maintain a patent airway until endotracheal intubation can be attempted in a controlled and equipped area of the hospital [19]. Patients with jaw and zygomatic arch injuries often have trismus. Although the trismus will resolve with the administration of neuromuscular blocking agents, pre-induction assessment of airway anatomy may be difficult [11]. Rapid sequence intubation with cervical in-line immobilization is the preferred method of intubating the trachea of the trauma patients. Both maxillary and mandibular fractures will probably make mask ventilation more difficult. However, mandibular fractures will make intubation easier because of loss of skeletal resistance to direct laryngoscopy.

Le Fort II and III fractures mandate oral intubation because of the intranasal damage. In the case of mandibular or Le Fort I fractures, if no trismus or mechanical problem exists, routine rapid-sequence tracheal intubation is the technique of choice [11,17]. If it is judged that direct laryngoscopy may be difficult, then any technique that will preserve spontaneous ventilation should be used; such as awake fiberoptic, retrograde, and laryngeal mask–guided intubation [17,20–22].

The use of blind nasal intubation in the presence of facial trauma is controversial [18]. The source of disagreement is multiple case reports of nasogastric tubes placed intracranially in the presence of base of skull fracture [23]. Cephalic placement of an endotracheal tube is rare because the tube is much less flexible [23–25]. No significant complications were identified in a retrospective evaluation of blind nasal intubation of 82 patients suffering facial fractures [24]. The same attitude can be found at the modification of the American Society of Anesthesiologists (ASA) difficult airway algorithm to trauma. In this modification, there are only 3 contraindications. Yet, there is no absolute dismissal of the technique in the presence of maxillofacial trauma [18]. This issue is well summarized in an editorial statement: "Rapid sequence induction is the cornerstone of modern emergency airway management. Nasotracheal intubation is not contraindicated in the presence of severe maxillofacial or skull injuries providing a proper technique is used" [25].

The struggle to intubate may waste precious time, compromise the patient's respiratory status, and elevate intracranial pressure. The use of laryngeal mask airway is very important technique as an adjunct when you cannot intubate or ventilate in these situations (ASA guidelines). Cricothyroidotomy is a useful alternative with a 90% success rate even in inexperienced hands [19]. Perhaps early cricothyroidotomy, rather than repeated multiple attempts to intubate, would result in less hypoxia and improved patient outcome. Emergency tracheotomy is not considered an appropriate method to establish emergency definitive airway because the procedure is lengthy and carries a significant rate of complications.

ASA difficult airway algorithm modification for trauma

The ASA Task Force on Difficult Airway Management presents guidelines for the management of the difficult airway (DA). The algorithm gives the physician a systematic approach to nonsurgical methods of ventilation before a surgical pathway is elected. However the ASA algorithm is only generally applicable to the trauma patient. The time taken to obtain nonsurgical airway control may not be in the best interest of the trauma patient in whom risk of hemorrhagic shock, aspiration, and head trauma often exist. Indeed, in cases of severe trauma, the crisis approach to management often precludes continuing with nonsurgical methods of airway ventilation, and a surgical airway is sometimes elected at a point in time before that which would be the case in other patient populations. Ultimately, it is clinical judgment that guides the path taken in obtaining airway control in trauma patients.

Recently a trial to modify the difficult airway algorithm to trauma was done [18]. Obviously, maxillofacial and neck trauma falls into the category of suspected difficult intubation. The key points in the modified algorithm are:

Stopping is seldom an option with trauma.
Surgical airway can be the first/best choice in *certain conditions*.
An awake ETT technique should be chosen in a DA patient providing the patient is cooperative, stable, and spontaneously ventilating.
If the patient is uncooperative/combative general anesthesia (GA) may need to be administered, but if the airway is difficult, spontaneous ventilation (SV) should be continued (if possible).

The DA algorithm modification for trauma defines invasive airway access as surgical/percutaneous tracheostomy as well as cricothyroidotomy [18]. It seems worth mentioning that many practitioners do not believe tracheostomy is a proper way to gain emergency control of the airway whether surgically or percutaneously [26].

Summary

Penetrating face and neck trauma is usually obvious, but blunt trauma mandates high index of suspicion to recognize its existence. Comprehensive understanding of the injury is mandatory to plan the best timing and method to secure the airway. If the airway is stable, it is prudent for the most experienced anesthesia provider to acquire airway control in a controlled setting with surgical personnel immediately available should a surgical airway be indicated. If any doubt exists as to the clinician's ability to secure the airway, it is better to use a technique that maintains patient spontaneous ventilation.

References

[1] Kadish H, Schunk J, Woodward GA. Blunt pediatric laryngotracheal trauma: case reports and review of the literature. Am J Emerg Med 1994;12:207–11.
[2] Atkins BZ, Abbate S, Fisher SR, et al. Current management of laryngotracheal trauma. Case report and literature review. J Trauma 2004;56:185–90.
[3] Bhojani RA, Rosenbaum DH, Dickmen E, et al. Contemporary assessment of laryngotracheal trauma. J Thorac Cardiovasc Surg 2005;130:426–32.
[4] Kaufman HJ, Ciraulo DL, Burns P. Traumatic fracture of the hyoid bone: three case presentations of cardiorespiratory compromise secondary to missed diagnosis. Am Surg 1999;65: 877–80.
[5] Keogh IJ, Rowley H, Russel J. Critical airway compromise caused by neck hematoma. Clin Otolaryngol 2002;27:244–5.
[6] Vassiliu P, Baker J, Henderson S, et al. Aerodigestive injuries of the neck. Am Surg 2001;67: 75–9.
[7] Desjardins G, Varon AJ. Airway management for penetrating neck injuries: the Miami experience. Resuscitation 2001;48:71–5.
[8] Demetriades D, Velmahos GG, Asensio JA. Cervical pharyngotracheal and laryngotracheal injuries. World J Surg 2001;25:1044–8.
[9] van As AB, van Deurzen DFP, Verleisdonk EJMM. Gunshots to the neck: selective angiography as part of conservative management. Injury 2002;33:453–6.
[10] Hirshberg A, Wall MJ, Johnston RH, et al. Transcervical gunshot injuries. Am J Surg 1994; 167:309–12.
[11] Dutton RP, McCunn M. Anesthesia for trauma. In: Miller RD, editor. Miller's anesthesia. Philadelphia: Churchill Livingstone; 2005. p. 2451–9.
[12] Mussi A, Ambrogi MC, Ribechini A, et al. Acute major airway injuries: clinical features and management. Eur J Cardiothorac Surg 2001;20:46–52.
[13] Butler AP, Brennan PW, O'Rourke AK. Acute external laryngeal trauma—experience with 112 patients. Ann Otol Rhinol Laryngol 2005;114:361–8.
[14] Chen AY, Stewart MG, Raup G. Penetrating injuries of the face. Otolaryngol Head Neck Surg 1996;115:464–70.
[15] Lynham AJ, Hirst JP, Cosson JA, et al. Emergency department management of maxillofacial trauma. Emerg Med Australas 2004;16:7–12.
[16] Merrit RM, Williams MF. Cervical spine injury complicating facial trauma: incidence and management. Am J Otolaryngol 1997;18:235–8.
[17] Chesshire N, Knight DJW. The anaesthetic management of facial trauma and fractures. BJA–CEPD Reviews 2001;1(4):108–12.
[18] Wilson WC. Trauma: airway management. ASA difficult airway algorithm modified for trauma—and five common trauma intubation scenarios. ASA Newsletter; 2005;69:9–16.
[19] Leibovici D, Friedman B, Gofrit ON, et al. Prehospital cricothyroidotomy by physician. Am J Emerg Med 1997;15:91–3.
[20] Santhanagoppalan K, Chestnutt N, McBride G. Intubating LMA guided awake fiberoptic intubation in severe maxillofacial trauma. Can J Anaesth 2000;47:989–91.
[21] Patteson SK, Epps JL, Hall J. Simultaneous oral and nasal tracheal intubation utilizing a fiberoptic scope in a patient with facial trauma. J Clin Anesth 1996;8:258–9.
[22] Neal MR, Groves J, Gell IR, et al. Awake fiberoptic intubation in the semiprone position following facial trauma. Anaesthesia 1996;51:1053–4.
[23] Marlow TR, Goltra DD, Schabel SI. Intracranial placement of a nasotracheal tube after facial fracture: a rare complication. J Emerg Med 1997;15:187–91.

[24] Rosen CL, Wolfe RE, Chew SE, et al. Blind nasotracheal intubation in the presence of facial trauma. J Emerg Med 1997;15:141–5.

[25] Walls MW. Blind nasotracheal intubation in the presence of facial trauma—is it safe? J Emerg Med 1997;15:243–4.

[26] Mudler DS. Airway control. In: Moore EM, Mattox KL, Feliciano DV, editors. Trauma manual. 4th edition. New York: McGraw Hill; 2003. p. 70.

ELSEVIER
SAUNDERS

ANESTHESIOLOGY
CLINICS

Anesthesiology Clin
25 (2007) 13–21

The Critically Ill Injured Patient

Maurizio Cereda, MD[a,b], Yoram G. Weiss, MD[c],
Clifford S. Deutschman, MD[a,*]

[a]Department of Anesthesiology and Critical Care, University of Pennsylvania, HUP - 781A
Dulles, 3400 Spruce Street 4283, Philadelphia, PA 19104, USA
[b]Philadelphia VA Medical Center, University and Woodland Avenues,
Philadelphia, PA 19104, USA
[c]Department of Anesthesiology and Critical Care Medicine, Hadassah - Hebrew University
Medical Center, Kiryat Hadassah, P.O. Box 12000 J, Jerusalem 91120, Israel

Trauma patients admitted to the ICU frequently require surgical intervention. As a result, they require an extension of ICU treatment modalities to the operating room. Because these patients often have life-threatening problems (shock, acute respiratory distress syndrome [ARDS], sepsis) that do not relate directly to the operative procedure, it is essential that the anesthesiologist be aware of management strategies that are standard in critical care. However, management of these patients in the operating room is complicated by a series of practical problems. This article reviews the management of common respiratory and circulatory derangements that are likely to arise in the operative management of the trauma victim.

Damage control and abdominal compartment syndrome

Damage control is a strategy aimed at limiting the time that the acutely traumatized patient spends in the operating room. The goal of the initial abdominal operation is not to repair visceral injuries, but to control life-threatening hemorrhage, often by surgically packing injured areas. Subsequently, the patient is transported to the ICU for continuing hemodynamic resuscitation, correction of coagulopathies and of acidemia, and rewarming [1]. In abdominal trauma, damage control nearly always requires that the abdomen remain open. The abdominal viscera are protected with some type of dressing. The open management is used to facilitate re-exploration and to

* Corresponding author.
E-mail address: deutschcl@uphs.upenn.edu (C.S. Deutschman).

0889-8537/07/$ - see front matter © 2007 Elsevier Inc. All rights reserved.
doi:10.1016/j.atc.2006.11.008 *anesthesiology.theclinics.com*

prevent or treat abdominal compartment syndrome (ACS). ACS is a condition where a high intra-abdominal pressure (IAP) compromises the function of one or more organ systems [2]. The incidence of ACS in abdominal trauma has been reported to be as high as 36% [3] and has increased with the introduction of damage control [3]. The main risk factors for developing post-traumatic ACS are primary fascial closure, packing of hepatic injuries, massive fluid resuscitation, and the presence of pelvic injury [4]. Typically, ACS is associated with increases in airway pressures, acute renal failure, metabolic acidosis, and bowel hypoperfusion. The treatment of ACS is abdominal decompression and open management. This approach is continued until abdominal closure is possible. During open management, patients will require re-explorations, washouts, and repairs of visceral injuries. The hemodynamic management of the patient who has ACS can be challenging. Patients often are hemodynamically unstable and relatively hypovolemic. However, excessive volume loading can worsen edema of the bowel and of the abdominal wall, causing IAP to increase [5]. Thus, care must be taken when volume loading these patients; it requires careful management of ventilation and hemodynamics.

Care of the mechanically ventilated patient

Acute lung injury

Most critically ill trauma patients are ventilated mechanically and many have acute lung injury (ALI) or ARDS. These conditions can develop from direct pulmonary injuries (pulmonary contusion or laceration), toxic fume inhalation, blast injury, or gastric content aspiration. In other patients, lung injury may be induced by indirect injury mechanisms such as shock, massive resuscitation, transfusion, sepsis, or fat embolism.

Ventilator settings

Tidal volume and respiratory rate

For many years, tidal volume (VT) was set at supranormal values, such as 10 to 15 mL/kg body weight. However, recent studies have suggested that smaller VT (ie, 6 mL/kg ideal body weight) improve outcomes from ALI [6,7]. The rationale for these studies was provided by experimental evidence that ALI can also be caused by alveolar overdistension [8]. It is not known whether it is necessary to restrict VT in patients who do not have ALI. An observational study suggested that, among patients who do not initially have ALI, the probability of later developing this syndrome increases with the size of VT [9].

Low VT ventilation may require high respiratory rates to keep $Paco_2$ constant, which is especially true in patients who have ALI and ARDS. These individuals have elevated ventilatory demands because of high CO_2

production and increased alveolar dead space. However, increasing respiratory rates beyond 20 to 25 breaths per minute may not improve CO_2 excretion, and can lead to pulmonary hyperinflation [10]. Currently, it is considered acceptable to tolerate supranormal Pco_2 in patients who do not have contraindications to hypercapnia, such as elevated intracranial pressure or severe pulmonary hypertension.

Positive end-expiratory pressure and alveolar recruitment

Positive end-expiratory pressure (PEEP) is used in ALI to maintain alveolar recruitment and to reduce shunting of venous blood through nonventilated alveoli. The response to PEEP is variable, and seems to be related to the different causes of ALI [11]. PEEP decreases cardiac output by impairing venous return and ventricular filling, and also increases pulmonary vascular resistance, causing right ventricular failure [12].

Animal studies have shown the existence of alveolar instability when the lung is not recruited fully [13]. This phenomenon might worsen lung injury through mechanical stress and inflammatory activation [14]. Two clinical studies have attempted to demonstrate that PEEP improves outcomes of ALI by stabilizing alveolar recruitment. However, their results were discordant, likely because of differences in study design [7,15]. In the absence of definitive evidence, it is probably prudent to set PEEP pragmatically, trying to maximize oxygenation while minimizing side effects and complications. PEEP should not be increased beyond the level where the plateau pressure reaches 30–35 cm H_2O, unless VT can be decreased further. If hypoxemia has not improved at this point, the inspiratory/expiratory (I/E) ratio can be increased. This maneuver has the effect of increasing mean airway pressure, a variable that is related closely to arterial oxygenation. An I/E ratio higher than one (inverted ratio) is often used in severely hypoxemic patients.

In patients who continue to be hypoxic with high PEEP, recruitment maneuvers can be tried. These can be performed using "sighs" (periodic high volume breaths at a rate of 2 to 3 per minute [16]), or inflations to a pressure of 35 to 40 cm H_2O, maintained for 30 seconds to a minute [17]. Sighs require modified ventilators, but recruitment maneuvers can be performed manually, using a self-inflating bag or the anesthesia ventilator circuit. It is still unclear whether recruitment maneuvers have a permanent effect on oxygenation and outcomes [18].

Effect of intra-abdominal pressure on the respiratory system

Elevated IAP affects the mechanics of both the chest wall and the lung. These changes can be reversed with abdominal decompression [19]. During ACS, airway pressures typically are high because a high IAP causes the diaphragm to migrate cephalad, decreasing chest wall compliance [20]. However, lung volumes are decreased by high IAP, even in the presence of elevated airway pressures, because low chest wall compliance limits lung inflation. The safety limit for inspiratory pressures may need to be increased in these patients.

Diaphragm elevation caused by high IAP causes alveolar collapse in the lower lobes, and worsened oxygenation. Patients who have increased IAP are therefore likely to benefit from higher levels of PEEP [2,11].

Ventilatory management in the operating room

Mechanical ventilation of critically ill patients in the operating room can be complicated by the fact that the design of ICU ventilators is substantially different from that of anesthetic machines. Anesthesia ventilators often cannot provide the elevated minute volumes and airway pressures needed by ALI patients. ICU ventilators are single-circuit systems where gas from the wall supply enters the pneumatic system and is delivered to the patient through a servo-regulated inspiratory valve. The gas pressure in the pneumatic system, or "working pressure," is maintained at a high level to assure a high flow, even when patient airway pressures are high. Anesthesia machines are double-circuit systems, where the gas delivered to the patient is contained in a bellows. Inspiration is powered by pressurizing the gas in the chamber that contains the bellows. The presence of the bellows generates a high compression volume, which is the quota of inspiratory volume that does not reach the patient because it is "lost" in the cyclic compression of circuit gas. In ICU ventilators, compression volume is caused only by the circuit, and is usually 0.5 mL/cm H_2O [21]. Anesthetic ventilators operate with a compression volume as high as 6 to 12 mL/cm H_2O [22]. As a consequence, the VT and flow actually delivered to the patient become lower than the set values when airway pressures increases [22].

No guidelines suggest when an anesthesia ventilator is inadequate to provide support for a certain patient. Intuitively, patients requiring a high minute volume (ie, >10 l/min) with high peak airway pressures (>40 cm H_2O) likely will be harder to ventilate with an anesthesia machine. By comparing the results of in vitro measurements with the respiratory mechanics data of 200 ICU patients, Katz and colleagues [22] showed that a significant fraction of these patients exceeded the ventilator capabilities of commonly used ventilators. An anesthesia machine with servomechanisms that preserve delivery of VT at high pressures had a better performance than nonstandard machines. However, its performance was inferior to that of an ICU ventilator adapted for anesthetic gas delivery, because the latter had a single-circuit system.

When inadequate performance of the operating room ventilator is expected, an ICU ventilator should be used. The use of inhalational agents is not possible and an intravenous anesthesia should be chosen. Recently designed devices allow anesthetic delivery through an ICU ventilator using a system similar to a heat and moisture exchanger. Although these systems were designed originally for ICU sedation, they have been tested recently in the operative setting [23].

Choice of ventilator mode

The choice of ventilator mode is probably less important than applying the general principles outlined earlier. Some evidence indicates that ventilatory modes that partially support spontaneous breathing should be used when possible. Among these modes are pressure support ventilation and airway pressure release ventilation. Airway pressure release ventilation allows spontaneous breathing superimposed on a low rate of controlled breaths delivered at high pressure and very high I/E ratio. This mode has positive effects on gas exchange and decreases sedation requirements in trauma patients [24].

The patient who needs an operation should be maintained on the same mode and settings as in the ICU, which may be impossible, however, when a spontaneously breathing patient needs muscle relaxation, or when a certain mode is not available on the anesthesia ventilator. Care should be taken in assuring that similar mean airway pressures and minute volumes are maintained in the transition between different modes of ventilation, to avoid precipitation of hypoxemia and hypercapnia. Most anesthesia ventilators are volume controlled, but servo-controlled machines can deliver pressure-controlled ventilation. Evidence does not indicate a significant clinical difference between these two modes of ventilation.

Hemodynamic management

Patients who have chest or abdominal injuries often develop severe shock as a result of hypovolemia. Soon thereafter, appropriate resuscitation from hypovolemic shock gives rise to a vasodilatory state, the hypermetabolic phase of the response to injury. If this vasodilatory state becomes persistent, it is referred to as the systemic inflammatory response syndrome. Although this second phase of injury always occurs, some data suggest that the degree of vasodilatation and the subsequent development of systemic inflammatory response syndrome correlate with the extent of initial organ hypoperfusion-hypoxia, exposure to infection, and cytokine activation [25]. Therapy is, primarily, adequate fluid resuscitation to maintain adequate organ perfusion. However, overzealous fluid resuscitation may result in respiratory deterioration, which has significant impact on hemodynamics and may require intervention beyond simple fluid administration. Further, either fluid or vasopressor therapy may affect the function of other organs systems. Thus, careful monitoring of hemodynamics and an understanding of the end points of resuscitation are essential.

Monitoring the systemic circulation

Although data are lacking, severely injured patients may benefit from invasive monitoring to optimize fluid management, using either central venous pressure or pulmonary-artery catheters. However, the reliability of such measures has been called into question. Some experts believe that either transthoracic or transesophageal echocardiography may be more useful measures of fluid optimization than either central venous pressure or pulmonary capillary occlusion pressure (PAOP) [26]. Successive trans-esophageal echocardiography (TEE) seems to provide more accurate information on ventricular size than standard monitoring instruments, and recent data suggest that end diastolic volume is a better predictor of myocardial performance than PAOP, especially in ALI/ARDS patients or patients who have major abdominal injuries requiring elevated ventilatory pressures [27]. Airway pressures transmitted through the lung parenchyma may increase intrathoracic pressure, resulting in a falsely elevated PAOP that can mask a relatively hypovolemic state. Another approach that has been touted recently is pulse contour analysis. Use of infusion by way of a central vein allows determination of continuous cardiac output, and the combination of central and peripheral arterial waveforms permits calculation of intrathoracic blood volume and extravascular lung water. Significant mathematic assumptions are involved in this technique because the pressure waveform is obtained from a peripheral artery (radial or femoral) and not the aorta [28–30]. Although this approach is considered investigative in the United States, it is used routinely in many European centers.

Vasopressors to support the systemic circulation

The vasodilatory state that accompanies the response to injury or to systemic inflammatory response syndrome/sepsis is relatively nonspecific. As such, initial management involves administration of fluids to "fill the tank." At some point, however, this approach may become detrimental. For example, overadministration of fluids to a trauma patient may result in the development of ACS or may contribute to the pathology of ALI. Thus, alternatives to maintain organ perfusion must be sought. Vasopressor infusion is a mainstay.

Recent studies suggest that dilation in the splanchnic (visceral) circulation is more profound than that in the somatic (skeletal) circulation. Nonetheless, muscle is less vulnerable to ischemic injury than organs such as the brain, heart, kidney, gut, and liver. Therefore, vasoconstrictor agents that act primarily on the blood supply to the periphery are preferred. The choice of vasopressor agent is controversial [31–33]. Norepinephrine, a potent alpha and beta-1 agonist that has less effect on beta-2 receptors, has been proposed as the agent of choice [34]. Studies suggest that norepinephrine constricts the somatic circulation and redistributes blood volume to the viscera [35]. Recent studies indicate that dopamine, long a mainstay in trauma management, may be deleterious [36,37]. The highly nonspecific nature of this agent (it can stimulate a host of dopamine receptors as well as alpha, beta-1 and beta-2 receptors) makes it difficult to use. Epinephrine is a more potent beta-2 agonist than norepinephrine. Because beta-2 receptors lead to vasodilatation in the somatic circulation, this agent is less effective in translocating blood away from muscle and skin and toward organs [38,39]. Low doses of vasopressin may be sufficient to stimulate baroreceptors and raise the blood pressure. In sepsis or "chronic" critical illness, profound vasodilatation in the splanchnic circulation may result from depletion of vasopressin [40], and renal and hepatic insufficiency may impair elaboration of angiotensin-2 [32,41]. In vasodilatory shock, low doses (0.01–0.04 units/min) of vasopressin increase the mean arterial pressure through a V_1-mediated baroreceptor effect. The increased afterload is reflected in improved blood pressure, but may decrease the cardiac output. At these doses, vasopressin stimulates renal resorption of water by way of an aquaporin-2 effect, potentiates norepinephrine effects, and may improve renal function [42]. However, even at this relatively low dose, recent reports indicate stimulation of splanchnic V_2 receptors, resulting in vasoconstriction and possible intestinal ischemia. Above a dose of 0.04 U/min, splanchnic perfusion unquestionably is compromised. Therefore, the authors' approach is to start with a vasopressin dose of 0.01 U/min or less and avoid doses above 0.04 U/min.

Summary

This article attempted to present the problems that may be encountered in patients who have severe abdominal and lung injuries. The authors have presented current management concepts used in caring for these patients in the critical care setting. These management guidelines could serve the anesthetist faced with these patients in the operating room.

References

[1] Rotondo MF, Schwab CW, McGonigal MD, et al. 'Damage control': an approach for improved survival in exsanguinating penetrating abdominal injury. J Trauma 1993;35: 375–82 [discussion: 382–3].

[2] Malbrain ML. Abdominal pressure in the critically ill: measurement and clinical relevance. Intensive Care Med 1999;25:1453–8.

[3] Raeburn CD, Moore EE, Biffl WL, et al. The abdominal compartment syndrome is a morbid complication of postinjury damage control surgery. Am J Surg 2001;182:542–6.

[4] Ertel W, Oberholzer A, Platz A, et al. Incidence and clinical pattern of the abdominal compartment syndrome after "damage-control" laparotomy in 311 patients with severe abdominal and/or pelvic trauma. Crit Care Med 2000;28:1747–53.

[5] Mutoh T, Lamm WJ, Embree LJ, et al. Volume infusion produces abdominal distension, lung compression, and chest wall stiffening in pigs. J Appl Physiol 1992;72:575–82.

[6] The Acute Respiratory Distress Syndrome Network. Ventilation with lower tidal volumes as compared with traditional tidal volumes for acute lung injury and the acute respiratory distress syndrome. N Engl J Med 2000;342:1301–8.

[7] Amato MB, Barbas CS, Medeiros DM, et al. Effect of a protective-ventilation strategy on mortality in the acute respiratory distress syndrome. N Engl J Med 1998;338:347–54.

[8] Dreyfuss D, Saumon G. Ventilator-induced lung injury: lessons from experimental studies. Am J Respir Crit Care Med 1998;157:294–323.

[9] Gajic O, Dara SI, Mendez JL, et al. Ventilator-associated lung injury in patients with-out acute lung injury at the onset of mechanical ventilation. Crit Care Med 2004;32: 1817–24.

[10] Vieillard-Baron A, Prin S, Augarde R, et al. Increasing respiratory rate to improve CO_2 clearance during mechanical ventilation is not a panacea in acute respiratory failure. Crit Care Med 2002;30:1407–12.

[11] Gattinoni L, Pelosi P, Suter PM, et al. Acute respiratory distress syndrome caused by pulmo-nary and extrapulmonary disease. Different syndromes? Am J Respir Crit Care Med 1998; 158:3–11.

[12] Vieillard-Baron A, Jardin F. Why protect the right ventricle in patients with acute respira-tory distress syndrome? Curr Opin Crit Care 2003;9:15–21.

[13] McCann UG 2nd, Schiller HJ, Carney DE, et al. Visual validation of the mechanical stabi-lizing effects of positive end-expiratory pressure at the alveolar level. J Surg Res 2001;99: 335–42.

[14] Chu EK, Whitehead T, Slutsky AS. Effects of cyclic opening and closing at low- and high-volume ventilation on bronchoalveolar lavage cytokines. Crit Care Med 2004;32:168–74.

[15] Brower RG, Lanken PN, MacIntyre N, et al. Higher versus lower positive end-expiratory pressures in patients with the acute respiratory distress syndrome. N Engl J Med 2004; 351:327–36.

[16] Pelosi P, Cadringher P, Bottino N, et al. Sigh in acute respiratory distress syndrome. Am J Respir Crit Care Med 1999;159:872–80.

[17] Grasso S, Mascia L, Del Turco M, et al. Effects of recruiting maneuvers in patients with acute respiratory distress syndrome ventilated with protective ventilatory strategy. Anesthesiology 2002;96:795–802.

[18] Brower RG, Morris A, MacIntyre N, et al. Effects of recruitment maneuvers in patients with acute lung injury and acute respiratory distress syndrome ventilated with high positive end-expiratory pressure. Crit Care Med 2003;31:2592–7.

[19] Ranieri VM, Brienza N, Santostasi S, et al. Impairment of lung and chest wall mechanics in patients with acute respiratory distress syndrome: role of abdominal distension. Am J Respir Crit Care Med 1997;156:1082–91.

[20] Mutoh T, Lamm WJ, Embree LJ, et al. Abdominal distension alters regional pleural pres-sures and chest wall mechanics in pigs in vivo. J Appl Physiol 1991;70:2611–8.

[21] Kacmarek RM, Hess D. Basic principles of ventilator machinery. In: Tobin MJ, editor. Principles and practice of mechanical ventilation. vol. 1. New York: Mc Graw Hill; 1994. p. 65–110.

[22] Katz JA, Kallet RH, Alonso JA, et al. Improved flow and pressure capabilities of the datex-ohmeda SmartVent anesthesia ventilator. J Clin Anesth 2000;12:40–7.

[23] Tempia A, Olivei MC, Calza E, et al. The anesthetic conserving device compared with con-ventional circle system used under different flow conditions for inhaled anesthesia. Anesth Analg 2003;96:1056–61.

[24] Putensen C, Zech S, Wrigge H, et al. Long-term effects of spontaneous breathing during ven-tilatory support in patients with acute lung injury. Am J Respir Crit Care Med 2001;164: 43–9.

[25] Keel M, Trentz O. Pathophysiology of polytrauma. Injury 2005;36:691–709.

[26] Boldt J. Clinical review: hemodynamic monitoring in the intensive care unit. Crit Care 2002; 6:52–9.

[27] Weiss YG, Pollak A, Gilon D. Transesophageal echocardiography in critical care medicine. Curr Opin Crit Care 1997;3:232–7.

[28] Berton C, Cholley B. Equipment review: new techniques for cardiac output measurement—oesophageal doppler, fick principle using carbon dioxide, and pulse contour analysis. Crit Care 2002;6:216–21.

[29] Bellomo R, Uchino S. Cardiovascular monitoring tools: use and misuse. Curr Opin Crit Care 2003;9:225–9.

[30] Sakka SG, Klein M, Reinhart K, et al. Prognostic value of extravascular lung water in critically ill patients. Chest 2002;122:2080–6.
[31] Krejci V, Hiltebrand LB, Sigurdsson GH. Effects of epinephrine, norepinephrine, and phenylephrine on microcirculatory blood flow in the gastrointestinal tract in sepsis. Crit Care Med 2006;34:1456–63.
[32] Treggiari MM, Romand JA, Burgener D, et al. Effect of increasing norepinephrine dosage on regional blood flow in a porcine model of endotoxin shock. Crit Care Med 2002;30: 1334–9.
[33] Reinelt H, Radermacher P, Kiefer P, et al. Impact of exogenous beta-adrenergic receptor stimulation on hepatosplanchnic oxygen kinetics and metabolic activity in septic shock. Crit Care Med 1999;27:325–31.
[34] Reinhart K, Sakka SG, Meier-Hellmann A. Haemodynamic management of a patient with septic shock. Eur J Anaesthesiol 2000;17:6–17.
[35] Hannemann L, Reinhart K, Grenzer O, et al. Comparison of dopamine to dobutamine and norepinephrine for oxygen delivery and uptake in septic shock. Crit Care Med 1995;23: 1962–70.
[36] Ma P, Danner RL. The many faces of sepsis-induced vascular failure. Crit Care Med 2002; 30:947–9.
[37] Segal JM, Phang PT, Walley KR. Low-dose dopamine hastens onset of gut ischemia in a porcine model of hemorrhagic shock. J Appl Physiol 1992;73:1159–64.
[38] Meier-Hellmann A, Reinhart K, Bredle DL, et al. Epinephrine impairs splanchnic perfusion in septic shock. Crit Care Med 1997;25:399–404.
[39] Sakr Y, Reinhart K, Vincent JL, et al. Does dopamine administration in shock influence outcome? Results of the sepsis occurrence in acutely ill patients (SOAP) study. Crit Care Med 2006;34:589–97.
[40] Landry DW, Levin HR, Gallant EM, et al. Vasopressin deficiency contributes to the vasodilation of septic shock. Circulation 1997;95:1122–5.
[41] Bastien O, Piriou V, Aouifi A, et al. Effects of dopexamine on blood flow in multiple splanchnic sites measured by laser doppler velocimetry in rabbits undergoing cardiopulmonary bypass. Br J Anaesth 1999;82:104–9.
[42] den Ouden DT, Meinders AE. Vasopressin: physiology and clinical use in patients with vasodilatory shock: a review. Neth J Med 2005;63:4–13.

ELSEVIER
SAUNDERS

Anesthesiology Clin
25 (2007) 23–34

ANESTHESIOLOGY
CLINICS

Current Concepts in Hemorrhagic Shock

Richard P. Dutton, MD, MBA[a,b,*]

[a]*University of Maryland School of Medicine,*
22 South Greene Street, Baltimore, MD 21201, USA
[b]*Division of Trauma Anesthesiology, R Adams Cowley Shock Trauma Center, University*
of Maryland Medical System, 22 South Greene Street, Baltimore, MD 21201, USA

Pathophysiology of hemorrhagic shock

Loss of intravascular volume triggers a predictable systemic response, mediated by both local vascular signaling and the neuroendocrine system [1]. Decreased filling pressures in the heart result in a decrease in cardiac output, in accordance with Starling's Law. Vasoconstriction of ischemia-tolerant vascular beds (eg, skin, muscle, gut) allows preservation of flow to organs that depend on a continuous supply of oxygen, principally the heart and the brain. Vasoconstriction is triggered by reduced blood pressure, pain, and cortical perception of injury. In injured tissue, local mediators act to constrict blood flow and reduce bleeding. Central sympathetic outflow is increased and parasympathetic flow is decreased, leading to an increase in heart rate and contractility. Adrenal stimulation results in the "fight or flight" response, with increased levels of circulating epinephrine.

Persistent hypoperfusion leads to cellular death and organ system failure. Cells that lose nutrient blood flow undergo necrotic cell death. Other cells undergo apoptosis, or "programmed cell death," sacrificing themselves in the face of insufficient resources. Cells in many organ systems have the ability to hibernate. Cells in the renal cortex, for example, stop filtering fluid at a level of ischemia less than that which causes necrosis.

Shock is more than a transient failure in oxygen supply, but also the systemic disease that follows [2]. Cells in the liver and gut may remain ischemic after flow is reestablished in the macrocirculation, because of the occlusion of capillary networks caused by edema [3]. This "no-reflow" phenomenon

---

* Division of Trauma Anesthesiology, R Adams Cowley Shock Trauma Center, University of Maryland Medical System, 22 South Greene Street, Baltimore, MD 21201.
E-mail address: rdutton@umaryland.edu

doi:10.1016/j.atc.2006.11.007

persists even after cardiac output is normalized. Reperfusion following hemorrhagic shock releases toxic mediators into the circulation; these mediators are potent immune modulators. Even short periods of relatively minor ischemia can trigger a cascade of cellular signaling and response that results in organ system failure (Fig. 1).

The consequences of ischemia first become apparent in the less critical organs. Skin and muscle cells become anaerobic, producing lactic acid. Organs of the splanchnic circulation hibernate (peristalsis and renal filtering cease) and then suffer cellular damage, progressing to organ system failure. Hypoperfusion of the liver results in decreased glucose availability, loss of clotting factors, and, eventually, cell death [4]. Intestinal mucosal cells lose the ability to transport nutrients; if ischemia persists, the barrier function of the gut is lost, and translocation of bacteria occurs from the intestinal lumen into the portal circulation.

The lungs are the downstream filter for toxic metabolites, inflammatory mediators released by ischemic cells, and translocated bacteria from the gut. The lungs are also the sentinel organ for the development of multiple organ system failure. The acute respiratory distress syndrome, occurring after hemorrhagic shock, was first described in the 1960s as "Da Nang lung" [5]. Pulmonary failure develops over 1 to 3 days following severe trauma, is exacerbated by ventilator-associated pneumonia, and may require weeks of supportive care to resolve. Increased pulmonary resistance may lead to right-heart failure, even in young patients.

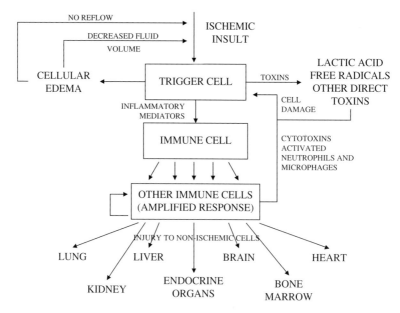

Fig. 1. The shock "cascade."

Symptoms of shock

Symptoms of shock are shown in Box 1. Vital signs do not reflect the quantity of hemorrhage accurately! Fit, young patients may lose 40% of their blood volume before the systolic blood pressure (SBP) drops below 100 mmHg, whereas the elderly may become hypotensive with volume loss of as little as 10% [6]. Hemorrhaging trauma patients are intensely vasoconstricted, and may suffer from end-organ ischemia even with a normal SBP [7]. Metabolic acidosis revealed by arterial blood gas measurement is the gold standard diagnostic test. Noninvasive monitors to diagnose shock are under development, as shown in Table 1.

Acute, fatal hemorrhagic shock is characterized by progressive metabolic acidosis, coagulopathy, and hypothermia (the lethal triad), followed by circulatory system failure [8]. Inappropriate vasodilatation results from loss of energy reserves in the vascular endothelium. Shock is seldom reversible at

---

Box 1. Signs and symptoms of hemorrhagic shock

Appearance
Pale, diaphoretic

Injuries
Open wounds, bruising, or bony instability consistent with
   blood loss

Mental status
Progressive deterioration from normal to agitated to lethargic
   to comatose

Vital signs
Decreased SBP (<100 mmHg), narrow pulse pressure,
   tachycardia, tachypnea, nonfunctional pulse oximeter,
   progressive hypothermia

Pulses
Diminished or absent, poor capillary refill

Renal
Diminished urine output

Laboratory
Decreased pH, abnormal base deficit, elevated lactate, elevated
   osmolarity, elevated prothrombin time (PT)

Response
Increased SBP with fluid administration (fluid responsiveness),
   exaggerated decrease with analgesics or sedatives

Table 1
Noninvasive shock monitors currently under development

Monitoring technology	Description	Comment
Gastric tonometry	Gastric pH reflects mucosal perfusion	Requires long calibration time; approved, but not commonly used
Sublingual capnometry	Sublingual pH easier to access than gastric; same correlation with perfusion	Faster than gastric tonometry, but still somewhat cumbersome
Near-infrared tissue oximetry	Reflectance oximetry of deltoid or thenar muscle bed	Approved and used in some ICUs; not yet proven in early shock management
Beat-to-beat heart rate variability	Analysis of EKG signal processed to determine sympathetic/parasympathetic balance	Encouraging preliminary results; needs more study in early patients who have severe hemorrhage
Acoustic arterial flow analysis	Compares vascular acoustic "signature" to determine degree of vasoconstriction	Not yet commercially available

this stage, even with massive transfusion. If perfusion is restored before this point, the ultimate outcome will depend on the total "dose" of shock (the depth and duration of hypoperfusion), the patient's underlying physiologic reserve, and the details of medical management.

System-specific actions to control hemorrhage

Table 2 shows the five compartments of the body into which significant intravascular volume can be lost [9]. Successful resuscitation is unlikely in the absence of hemostasis. Anatomic control of bleeding is the single most important step in resuscitation from hemorrhagic shock. Exsanguination to the environment ("the street") is easiest to diagnose, and is treated by direct pressure on the bleeding wound. By itself, external bleeding is seldom life-threatening. In the presence of other injuries, however, "a little scalp bleeding" may be overlooked, especially if it occurs from rebleeding caused by increased blood pressure and clotting factor dilution.

Bleeding into long-bone compartments is substantial at the time of injury, but ongoing hemorrhage is rare. Vasoconstriction in the periphery and tamponade in closed fascial compartments limit blood loss. Exceptions are open fractures and direct injury to major arteries. Opening of the fascia, disruption of periosseous clot, and blood dilution with intravenous fluids contribute to rebleeding at the time of surgical repair. It is wise to complete resuscitation, secure vascular access, and ensure the availability of blood products before definitive repair is attempted.

Injury to the lung causes low-pressure bleeding that usually stops spontaneously. Management is by placement of a tube thoracostomy, which allows

Table 2
Potential sites of exsanguination in the unstable trauma patient

Site of bleeding	Diagnostic modality
Chest	Physical examination (breath sounds, bruises, or abrasions)
	Chest radiograph
	Thoracostomy tube output
	CT scan
Abdomen	Physical examination (distention, pain)
	Ultrasound (FAST)
	CT with contrast
	Peritoneal lavage
Retroperitoneum	Physical examination (unstable pelvic ring)
	Pelvic radiograph
	CT with contrast
	Angiography
Long bones	Physical examination
	Plain radiographs
Outside the body	Medic's or bystander's report
	Physical examination

Abbreviation: FAST, Focused Assessment by Sonography in Trauma.

for drainage and quantification of hemorrhage, underwater seal of the pleural space, and application of continuous suction. Fewer than 15% of patients will require emergent surgical exploration, typically as the result of bleeding from the hilum of the lung or from a lacerated intercostal artery [10]. Initial blood loss in excess of 1 L, or ongoing bleeding greater than 200 mL/hour, should prompt surgical exploration. Traumatic aortic rupture results from high-energy blunt trauma, and represents a spectrum of disease, from minor intimal disruption to complete transection. Tamponade by surrounding structures may prevent exsanguination into the left pleural space, allowing a window of opportunity for diagnosis and surgical therapy [11]. The use of angiographic stent grafting will soon become the standard of care for these injuries.

Hemorrhage in the mediastinum is a true emergency, and a successful outcome depends on rapid surgical management. Shock develops from cardiac tamponade, and patients require emergent pericardotomy; if the underlying cardiac or vascular injury can be controlled, and a perfusing blood pressure restored, the patient will often recover.

Abdominal hemorrhage is diagnosed by ultrasound: the Focused Assessment by Sonography for Trauma examination. Hemorrhage may also be diagnosed by CT or by diagnostic peritoneal lavage. In the stable patient, CT followed by angiographic embolization of liver or splenic bleeding may allow for successful, nonoperative management. Hemorrhage in an unstable patient indicates emergent laparotomy. "Damage control surgery" is the concept of a swift initial operation focused only on control of hemorrhage, followed by re-exploration and definitive surgery after 24 to 48 hours of ICU stabilization [12].

Life-threatening retroperitoneal hemorrhage arises from injury to the venous plexus that lies on the inner surface of the sacrum. Patients who have posterior venous plexus bleeding are transient responders to initial fluid therapy. Physical examination reveals instability of the pelvis, and plain film radiography shows the fracture. Pelvic venous bleeding is not accessible surgically. Abdominal exploration in this setting may be counterproductive, because it releases tamponade of the retroperitoneal hematoma. Treatment is by urgent pelvic compression with a pelvic binder or external fixator to facilitate tamponade, followed by angiographic embolization of pelvic vessels and orthopedic stabilization of the sacroiliac joint [13].

Fluid resuscitation: strategy

Minimizing hypoperfusion and tissue ischemia would seem to dictate rapid volume resuscitation in the actively bleeding patient. Unfortunately, there are competing priorities. Before definitive hemostasis, vigorous fluid administration increases the rate of bleeding from injured vessels. Fluid administration raises cardiac output and increases blood pressure. Increased blood pressure counters local vasoconstrictive mechanisms and exerts greater force on fragile clots [14]. When isotonic crystalloids are used, dilution of the blood is inevitable, which reduces hematocrit (lowering oxygen carrying capacity) and reduces the concentration of clotting factors and platelets. Hypothermia is a strong possibility, contributing to the development of coagulopathy. Typically, crystalloid administration leads to a transient rise in blood pressure, followed by an increase in the rate of hemorrhage and a subsequent deterioration, which, in turn, begets further fluid administration, leading to the "bloody vicious cycle" of hypotension, fluid bolus, rebleeding, and deeper hypotension [15]. The Advanced Trauma Life Support (ATLS) curriculum recommends rapid administration of up to 2 L of crystalloid, followed by continued blood and crystalloid targeted to a normal pulse and blood pressure, but includes the following statement: "Aggressive and continued volume resuscitation is not a substitute for manual or operative control of hemorrhage" [9].

Laboratory evidence supporting a lower blood pressure target during active bleeding is substantial. In 1965, Shaftan [16] demonstrated that blood loss from a femoral artery injury in dogs was greatest in quantity and most prolonged when fluids or vasopressors were given, and least and shortest when either resuscitation was withheld or vasodilators were administered. Swine [14] and rat [17] models of uncontrolled hemorrhage have demonstrated that optimal oxygen delivery and survival is achieved in animals resuscitated to a lower target blood pressure. A consensus conference in 1993 summarized the available animal data, and advocated human trials of deliberate hypotensive resuscitation for patients who have active hemorrhage [18].

Two such trials have been conducted. The first included 600 hypotensive victims of penetrating thoracoabdominal trauma [19]. Patients were randomized to standard care (two large bore IVs, fluid administration to maintain SBP>100) or to fluid restriction (no IV fluids), and this therapy was continued to the operating room. Patients in the no-fluids group received less fluid than those in the standard care group, but had a similar SBP. Survival in the no-fluids group was 60%, versus 54% in the standard care group ($P = .04$). Despite the positive result of this trial, it was criticized for its all-or-none approach, its restriction to penetrating trauma patients, and its failure to continue fluid restriction into the operative period.

The results of this trial are supported by other data. Patients receiving fluids by way of a rapid infusion system were found retrospectively to do poorly, compared with historical controls [20]. In a prospective trial, patients presenting in hemorrhagic shock were randomized to conventional treatment (SBP>100) or restricted treatment (SBP>80), and this therapy was continued until definitive control of hemorrhage [21]. The rate of mortality was not different (4 of 55 patients in each group), but hemorrhage was controlled more rapidly in the low-pressure group.

A consensus approach to early resuscitation is summarized in Box 2. The priority is to identify the patient who is bleeding actively. Intubation and mechanical ventilation allow for better analgesia and more rapid transition to CT, operating room, and angiography. Blood pressure is kept low, with an emphasis on preserving blood composition.

The hemostatic moment is easy to identify. Even without exogenous fluid administration, a hypovolemic patient will "auto-resuscitate" if there is no ongoing blood loss [21]. At this point, the targets for resuscitation shift to the more familiar list in Box 3, with the administration of fluids to achieve

---

Box 2. Goals for early resuscitation (prior to definitive control of hemorrhage)

Control of airway and ventilation
Expeditious control of hemorrhage
SBP 80–100 mmHg
Blood composition
• Limited use of crystalloid fluid
• Hematocrit 25%–30%, with early administration of red blood cells (RBCs) (including uncrossmatched Type O)
• Early use of plasma to maintain normal clotting studies
• Possible use of cryoprecipitate and/or Factor VIIa if patient is already coagulopathic
• Platelet count >50,000
• Ionized calcium monitored and treated
Maintained core temperature of >35°C
Gradual conversion to deep general anesthesia

Box 3. Goals for late resuscitation (after definitive control of hemorrhage)

Complete resuscitation is achieved by titrated administration of fluids until the following parameters are met
Normal or hyperdynamic vital signs
Hematocrit >20% (transfusion threshold determined by patient's age)
Normal serum electrolytes
Normal coagulation function, platelet count of at least 50,000
Restoration of adequate microvascular perfusion, as indicated by
- pH = 7.40 with normal base deficit
- Normalized serum lactate
- Normal mixed venous oxygenation
- Normal or high cardiac output
Normal urine output

---

normal vital signs and to restore perfusion in the microcirculation. Trauma patients may normalize their blood pressure while still hypovolemic. This "occult hypoperfusion" carries a high risk for subsequent organ system failure, sepsis, and death [22]. Although normal pH is a good indicator of adequate fluid volume, serum lactate level is a better indicator of the depth and duration of shock. The rate at which shock patients normalize lactate is correlated strongly with outcome [7]. Patients who do not clear lactate with post-hemorrhage fluid loading are suspicious for ongoing hemorrhage or occult myocardial dysfunction, and should be assessed further. Measurement of cardiac output is indicated, with judicious use of inotropic agents in patients who do not respond to adequate preload [23].

Fluid resuscitation: component therapy

Fluid resuscitation must restore intravascular volume, oxygen delivery, and hemostatic capability. Fresh whole blood is the ideal fluid for victims of serious hemorrhagic trauma, because it meets these goals with the least potential for side effects [24]. Except in certain military settings, this therapy is not available in the United States. "Component therapy" refers to the practice of fractionating units of donated whole blood into separate units of red cells, plasma, and platelets.

Many trauma patients do not need blood products at all. Isotonic crystalloid administration replaces the deficit in intravascular volume associated with acute hemorrhage, and produces an increase in cardiac output. In hemostatic patients this may be sufficient, but in actively bleeding patients the benefit is transient. It is important to identify the transient responder early.

Whether using deliberate hypotension or not, use of crystalloid as the primary resuscitative fluid causes a drop in hematocrit and clotting factor concentrate. Hypotension persisting or returning after an initial bolus of crystalloid is a strong indicator for RBC transfusion.

Colloid solutions are also used during resuscitation, especially in European trauma systems. Isotonic crystalloids equilibrate rapidly across all fluid compartments, leaving as little as 11% in the intravascular space 60 minutes after administration [25]; however, colloids are highly osmotic, and will draw free fluid into the circulation. The immediate effect of colloid on vascular volume, cardiac output, and blood pressure is greater than the effect of a similar dose of crystalloid. In some (nonbleeding) patients, the more rapid restoration of perfusion is a benefit, whereas in others, the rapid increase in blood pressure contributes to rebleeding.

Preservation of oxygen delivery is the goal of early resuscitation. Most severely injured patients requires transfusion of heterologous blood. RBC administration should begin as soon as severe hemorrhagic shock is diagnosed, without waiting for laboratory measures. Because the unresuscitated patient is losing whole blood, the hemoglobin concentration and hematocrit will not change until substantial fluid shifts have occurred. Systemic acidosis, indicated by decreased pH, elevated lactate, or abnormal base deficit, is a sensitive indicator of the need for transfusion, but even these tests take time. Waiting to begin transfusion until the patient is demonstrably anemic creates a perfusion deficit that makes later resuscitation more difficult. Early use of RBCs limits the dilutional effects of crystalloid administration, and supports oxygen delivery to ischemic tissues. Unstable patients who have active ongoing hemorrhage are resuscitated with a "whole blood" solution: equal parts of RBCs, plasma, and platelets. Even with this mixture, it is difficult to restore normal blood composition because of anticoagulant dilution and losses during storage (Table 3). Many trauma centers maintain a supply of "universal donor" type-O

Table 3
Donated versus delivered composition of blood products

Component	When donated	After fractionation	When administered to a patient in a 1:1:1 ratio
Total volume	500 mL	700 mL	700 mL
Red blood cells	Hematocrit = 45%	450 mL Hematocrit = 55%	Hematocrit = 28%
Plasma	Clotting factor activity = 100%	200 mL Activity = 90%	Activity = 65%
Platelets	Approx. 300,000/ hpf	50 mL	Approximately 65,000/hpf

Donated whole blood is diluted with an anticoagulant solution and then centrifuged and fractionated, resulting in the loss of potency when that unit is "reconstituted."

blood on hand for immediate transfusion. The use of uncrossmatched type-O RBCs in this setting is highly efficacious [26].

Clotting function is critical in the patient who has ongoing hemorrhagic shock. Plasma administration to support normal prothrombin time (PT) becomes necessary with acute blood loss of 30% to 40% of the normal blood volume (1500–2000 mL), whereas platelets are needed shortly thereafter. Patients requiring more than 10 units of RBC transfusion are likely to receive comparable amounts of plasma and platelets [27]. Because of the logistic barriers involved in administering blood products, it is advisable to order plasma and platelets early in resuscitation.

Patients who have severe shock, and those bleeding very rapidly, may be coagulopathic when first encountered. It is seldom possible to reverse coagulopathy once it has started. Interest is developing in a "jump-start" approach to achieve hemostasis in acutely coagulopathic patients. This approach consists of the rapid administration of concentrated fibrinogen (in the form of 8–10 units of cryoprecipitate), platelets (1–2 pheresis units), and recombinant clotting factor VIIa (FVIIa; 90 mcg/kg). Therapy with FVIIa in nonhemophiliacs is not approved by the Food and Drug Administration, and carries an unknown risk of provoking a thromboembolic complication [28], but has been reported to be a successful adjunctive therapy [29].

Rapid transfusion may lead to the development of hypocalcemia, caused by the binding of calcium by the anticoagulant in stored blood components. This "citrate intoxication" is diagnosed by decreased ionized calcium, and is treated by calcium administration to preserve cardiac contractile function [30]. Empiric calcium therapy should be considered in the hypotensive patient who is receiving blood quickly. Abnormalities in other electrolytes are less likely during massive resuscitation, although hyperkalemia can result from ongoing acidosis, wash-out of ischemic vascular beds, and lysis of transfused RBCs.

Hypothermia improves outcomes in carefully controlled animal models of shock, but is not recommended for humans [31]. Coagulation is affected strongly by temperature, and hypothermia may lead to increased hemorrhage. The use of fluid warming systems, warmed operating rooms, and forced hot air blankets is recommended strongly.

Controversies

Older patients have decreased physiologic reserve, compared with younger patients. Blood loss will produce hypotension earlier, and a smaller dose of shock will lead to organ system dysfunction. Diagnostic and therapeutic precision is important in this population, as is a high index of suspicion for medical conditions that predate the trauma. One of these is the routine use of anticoagulant medications such as aspirin, clopidogrel, or coumadin. Providers must seek medical history from the patient's family, and act quickly to reverse acquired coagulopathies with plasma, platelets, or factor

VIIa [32]. A higher blood pressure target is appropriate in patients who have hypertension at baseline.

Traumatic brain injury per se does not contribute to shock, but it does have a profound effect on outcome [33]. Deliberate hypotension in hemorrhaging patients who have traumatic brain injury is controversial, because of the known association between hypotensive episodes and worsened outcomes from traumatic brain injury. Limited laboratory data indicate that control of hemorrhage is still the most critical variable, and that a lower than normal blood pressure target is appropriate if death from hemorrhage is the greater risk [34].

Summary

Hemorrhagic shock is triggered by hypoperfusion caused by blood loss, but perpetuated by ongoing systemic responses. Current treatment concepts focus on diagnosis by evidence of tissue ischemia (rather than abnormal vital signs), rapid anatomic control of hemorrhage, facilitation of hemostasis, and maintenance of blood composition. Future advances will be driven by the ability to manipulate clotting directly, by improved monitoring of tissue perfusion, and by an understanding of the inflammatory consequences of shock and how best to manage them.

References

[1] Runciman WB, Sjowronski GA. Pathophysiology of haemorrhagic shock. Anaesth Intensive Care 1984;12:193–205.

[2] Peitzman AB. Hypovolemic shock. In: Pinsky MR, Dhainaut JFA, editors. Pathophysiologic foundations of critical care. Baltimore (MD): Williams & Wilkins; 1993. p. 161–9.

[3] Chun K, Zhang J, Biewer J, et al. Microcirculatory failure determines lethal hepatocyte injury in ischemic-reperfused rat livers. Shock 1994;1:3–9.

[4] Peitzman AB, Corbett WA, Shires GT III, et al. Cellular function in liver and muscle during hemorrhagic shock in primates. Surg Gynecol Obstet 1985;161:419–24.

[5] Eiseman B. Pulmonary effects of nonthoracic trauma. J Trauma 1968;8:649–50.

[6] Committee on Trauma, American College of Surgeons. Advanced trauma life support program for doctors. Chicago: American College of Surgeons; 1997.

[7] Abramson D, Scalea TM, Hitchcock R, et al. Lactate clearance and survival following injury. J Trauma 1993;35:584–8.

[8] Moore EE. Staged laparotomy for the hypothermia, acidosis, coagulopathy syndrome. Am J Surg 1996;72:405–10.

[9] Scalea TM, Henry SM. Assessment and initial management in the trauma patient. Problems in Anesthesia 2001;13:271–8.

[10] Wall MJ, Storey JH, Mattox K. "Indications for thoracotomy." In: Mattox K, Feliciano DV, Moore EE, editors. Trauma, 4th edition. New York: McGraw-Hill; 2000. p. 475.

[11] Cowley RA, Turney SZ, Hankins JR, et al. Rupture of thoracic aorta caused by blunt trauma. J Thorac Cardiovasc Surg 1990;100:652–61.

[12] Rotondo MF, Schwab CW, McGonigal MD, et al. 'Damage control': an approach for improved survival in exsanguinating penetrating abdominal injury. J Trauma 1993;35:375–82.

[13] Olson SA, Burgess A. Classification and initial management of patients with unstable pelvic ring injuries. Instr Course Lect. 2005;54:383–93.

[14] Stern A, Dronen SC, Birrer P, et al. Effect of blood pressure on haemorrhagic volume in a near-fatal haemorrhage model incorporating a vascular injury. Ann Emerg Med 1993; 22:155–63.

[15] Moore FA, McKinley BA, Moore EE. The next generation in shock resuscitation. Lancet. 2004;363:1988–96.

[16] Shaftan GW, Chiu C, Dennis C, et al. Fundamentals of physiologic control of arterial hemorrhage. Surgery 1965;58:851–6.

[17] Capone A, Safar P, Stezoski SW, et al. Uncontrolled hemorrhagic shock outcome model in rats. Resuscitation 1995;29:143–52.

[18] Shoemaker WC, Peitzman AB, Bellamy R, et al. Resuscitation from severe hemorrhage. Crit Care Med 1996;24:S12–23.

[19] Bickell WH, Wall MJ, Pepe PE, et al. Immediate versus delayed resuscitation for hypotensive patients with penetrating torso injuries. N Engl J Med 1994;331:1105–9.

[20] Hambly PR, Dutton RP. Excess mortality associated with the use of a rapid infusion system at a level 1 trauma center. Resuscitation 1996;31:127–33.

[21] Dutton RP, Mackenzie CF, Scalea TM. Hypotensive resuscitation during active hemorrhage: impact on in-hospital mortality. J Trauma 2002;52:1141–6.

[22] Blow O, Magliore L, Claridge JA, et al. The golden hour and the silver day: detection and correction of occult hypoperfusion within 24 hours improves outcome from major trauma. J Trauma 1999;47:964–9.

[23] Abou-Khalil B, Scalea TM, Trooskin SZ, et al. Hemodynamic responses to shock in young trauma patients: need for invasive monitoring. Crit Care Med 1994;22:633–9.

[24] Rhee P, Koustova E, Alam HB. Searching for the optimal resuscitation method: recommendations for the initial fluid resuscitation of combat casualties. J Trauma 2003;54(5 Suppl): S52–62.

[25] McIlroy DR, Kharasch ED. Acute intravascular volume expansion with rapidly administered crystalloid or colloid in the setting of moderate hypovolemia. Anesth Analg 2003;96: 1572–7.

[26] Dutton RP, Shih D, Edelman BB, et al. Safety of uncrossmatched type-O red cells for resuscitation from hemorrhagic shock. J Trauma 2005;59:1445–9.

[27] Como JJ, Dutton RP, Scalea TM, et al. Blood transfusion use rates in the care of acute trauma. Transfusion 2004;44:809–13.

[28] O'Connell KA, Wood JJ, Wise RP, et al. Thromboembolic adverse events after use of recombinant human coagulation factor VIIa. JAMA 2006;295:293–8.

[29] Dutton RP, McCunn M, Hyder M, et al. Factor VIIa for correction of traumatic coagulopathy. J Trauma 2004;57:709–19.

[30] Maitra SR, Geller ER, Pan W, et al. Altered cellular calcium regulation and hepatic glucose production during hemorrhagic shock. Circ Shock 1992;38:14–21.

[31] Dutton RP. Hypothermia and hemorrhage. In: Spiess BD, Spence RK, Shander A, editors. Perioperative transfusion medicine. 2nd edition. Philadelphia: Lippincott Williams & Wilkins; 2006. p. 481–6.

[32] Deveras RAE, Kessler CM. Reversal of warfarin-induced excessive anticoagulation with recombinant factor VII concentrate. Ann Intern Med 2002;137:884–8.

[33] Chestnut RM, Marshall LF, Klauber MR, et al. The role of secondary brain injury in determining outcome from severe head injury. J Trauma 1993;134:216–22.

[34] Novak L, Shackford SR, Bourguignon P, et al. Comparison of standard and alternative prehospital resuscitation in uncontrolled hemorrhagic shock and head injury. J Trauma 1999; 47:834–44.

ELSEVIER
SAUNDERS

ANESTHESIOLOGY
CLINICS

Anesthesiology Clin
25 (2007) 35–48

Nonsurgical Treatment of Major Bleeding

Rolf Rossaint, MD, PhD[a],*,
Jacques Duranteau, MD, PhD[b],
Philip F. Stahel, MD[c],
Donat R. Spahn, MD, FRCA[d]

[a]*Department of Anesthesiology, Aachen University, Pauwelsstr. 30, 52074 Aachen, Germany*
[b]*Department of Critical Care and Anesthesiology, University Paris XI, Bicêtre Hospital,
63 rue Gabriel Péri, Le Kremlin-Bicêtre, F-94276 Paris, France*
[c]*Department of Orthopedic Surgery, Denver Health Medical Center, University of Colorado
School of Medicine, 777 Bannock Street, Denver, CO 80204, USA*
[d]*Department of Anaesthesiology, University Hospital Lausanne, CHUV, rue du Bugnon 46,
CH-1011 Lausanne, Switzerland*

Trauma is a major cause of mortality worldwide, accounting for 5 million deaths per year [1,2] and representing a major socioeconomic burden to society because of losses in productivity and psychologic burden in grief and suffering [1].

Recent years have seen significant improvements in resuscitation of trauma patients. Uncontrolled bleeding remains a major challenge, being responsible for approximately 40% of trauma-related deaths [3–5]. Uncontrolled bleeding is regarded as the leading cause of preventable death following trauma [3–6].

Management of bleeding in the first hours after trauma is key in preventing death. For bleeding resulting from identifiable vascular damage, a combination of packing, damage-control surgery, external fixation, and angiographic embolization can be highly effective. Damage-control surgery (such as laparotomy) is aimed at increasing survival of severely injured patients by abbreviating surgical procedures and allowing early transfer of the patient to intensive care. It allows for tamponade and repair of some injured vessels, whereas external fixation can help control small venous

---

Dr. Rossaint and Dr. Spahn have received lecture sponsorship from Novo Nordisk.
* Corresponding author.
E-mail address: rossaint@post.rwth-aachen.de (R. Rossaint).

and cancellous bone bleeding. Because the focus of this article is nonsurgical management of major bleeding, these approaches to bleeding control are not discussed further but are reviewed extensively elsewhere [7–12]. Angiographic embolization is increasingly used in the early management of selected trauma patients and is reviewed briefly.

Although the combination of surgery, damage control, external fixation, and embolization may arrest bleeding resulting from vascular damage in some cases of traumatic injury, many patients who have major uncontrolled bleeding develop coagulopathic diffuse bleeding that requires other nonsurgical approaches to management. A state of coagulopathy poses unique challenges to the anesthetist and surgeon. As described, coagulopathy can result from a coalition of factors inherent to trauma and its management [4,13]. Blood component replacement therapy, although the mainstay of management for massive blood loss, cannot always restore the efficacy of the blood coagulation system, and the prevention and treatment of trauma-related coagulopathy may require correction of normal coagulation processes. Adjunctive use of fibrinogen may be tried to correct the coagulopathy associated with massive blood loss and its management, and recent studies suggest that adjunctive use of recombinant activated factor VII (rFVIIa; eptacog alpha, NovoSeven) may have a role in trauma hemostasis. This article considers new developments in the contemporary, nonsurgical, management of critical trauma bleeding.

Angiography and embolization

Although surgery is the cornerstone of bleeding control, transcatheter angiographic embolization (TAE) is an increasingly popular and highly effective means of controlling arterial bleeding in blunt trauma patients who have suffered solid organ injury or pelvic fracture, offering success rates as high as 90% [14–17]. The technique is applicable in the control of arterial bleeding [18–21]. For example, Fangio and colleagues [22] reported a 96% success rate in a series of 25 hemodynamically unstable patients who had pelvic injuries, and Hagiwara and colleagues [23] reported a successful outcome following TAE in 19 patients who had blunt multiple trauma who showed only a transient response to fluid resuscitation. In general, hemodynamically unstable patients should not undergo embolization, but, rather, surgical bleeding control.

Early use of embolization

It is generally agreed that angiography and embolization should be performed early after admission [24] because delays (> 3 hours) are reported to increase mortality from 17% to 75% [25]. There is debate, however, as to when angiographic embolization should be performed relative to external fixation or surgical interventions for bleeding control. Ideally, neither procedure would be delayed. In practice in most institutions, it is necessary to decide which should be performed first. A key consideration is whether the main cause of hemorrhage is venous bleeding (which may be effectively controlled by external fixation) or arterial bleeding (which may be controlled by surgery or angiographic embolization), and whether sources of bleeding can be predicted early.

The literature on embolization attests to the ongoing debate on how best to sequence management. Several studies have investigated whether the pattern of pelvic fracture, according to the Young and Burgess classification, is predictive of the potential requirement for acute embolization. Eastridge and colleagues [17] analyzed the medical records for 86 patients who had pelvic fractures (40 stable, 46 unstable) who required ongoing resuscitation and found that the mortality rate was higher for patients who had unstable fractures who underwent laparotomy first compared with those who underwent angiography first (60% versus 25%), suggesting that angiography should be considered before laparotomy in patients who have unstable fracture patterns. Sarin and colleagues [26], however, could not show a consistent correlation between order of angiography, external fixation, or laparotomy, and outcome. Another study, a retrospective case series of bleeding pelvic factures, found that all patients who remained hypotensive despite resuscitation demonstrated bleeding on diagnostic angiography. These authors therefore suggest that patients who do not show a sustained response to resuscitation should undergo angiography without delay, with external fixation performed subsequently [27].

The technique and its safety

Angiography is usually performed using a radiolucent material. An abdominal flush is performed to assess abdominal sites, followed by a pelvic flush and selective internal and external iliac artery runs [24]. Injuries requiring embolization present by extravasation of contrast, false aneurysms, or vasospasm. Embolization is then performed using steel coils for main arteries and branches, or with Gelfoam suspension for small branch bleeding sites. Angiography should then be repeated to check that bleeding has stopped, for new sites, and for evidence of ongoing bleeding.

Pelvic embolization is generally associated with minimal morbidity. There are reports, however, of necrosis of the distal colon and ureter, bladder necrosis, perineal wound sepsis [28], and ischemic damage of the gluteal muscle [29]. Risks should therefore be borne in mind when considering angiographic embolization.

The success of angiographic embolization, like surgery, is highly operator-dependent, and currently, not all centers dealing with trauma have 24-hour access to angiographic diagnostic and treatment facilities. Future studies are needed to guide clinical decision-making and clarify the optimal timing of embolization relative to traditional surgical control of bleeding in trauma.

Blood component replacement therapy

The resuscitation of trauma patients who have critical bleeding typically involves infusion of large volumes of crystalloid and colloid to restore tissue normoxia and correct tissue hypoperfusion, followed by use of blood and blood component transfusion in patients who are hemodynamically unstable, patients who have class III and IV hemorrhage (according to Advanced Trauma Life Support [ATLS] classification of shock), and patients who have uncontrolled ongoing sources of bleeding [7,30,31].

Although red blood cell (RBC) units help improve tissue oxygenation, they contain negligible amounts of platelets and coagulation factors. Consequently, in trauma patients who have bleeding described as nonsurgical (ie, cannot be controlled by conventional surgery, damage-control practices, fixation, or embolization and use of blood products), there is a need to adopt transfusion and hemostatic management strategies aimed at correcting coagulation deficits and the development of coagulopathy [32].

Coagulopathic diffuse bleeding in trauma

In trauma patients, normal coagulation capacity is often severely compromised. When coagulopathy is present with hypothermia and acidosis, the so-called "lethal triad" may ensue, leading to exsanguination and death [33]. Coagulopathy often occurs early postinjury, and predicts for significantly higher rates of mortality [13]. Patients who have an injury severity score (ISS) greater than 25, systolic blood pressure less than 70 mm Hg, acidosis (pH < 7.1), and hypothermia (temperature < 34°C) show an increased risk for developing coagulopathy [34].

The factors contributing to trauma coagulopathy are numerous and often compounding (Box 1) [32].

Box 1. Major causes and contributors to the development of coagulopathy in trauma patients [32]

- Blood loss
- Consumption of platelets and coagulation factors
- Dilution of platelets and coagulation factors
- Increased fibrinolysis
- Impaired functions of platelets and coagulation factors
- Coagulation-compromising effects of colloids
- Hypothermia
- Hypocalcemia

Data from Spahn DR, Rossaint R. Coagulopathy and blood component transfusion in trauma. Br J Anaesth 2005;95:130–9.

Blood loss is a major factor in trauma-associated coagulopathy (Fig. 1) [35–37]. In addition, there is often "consumption coagulopathy," whereby platelet and coagulation factors are depleted through the normal activation of the coagulation system in response to tissue damage or from abnormal activation of the coagulation system and fibrinolysis in response to prevailing anoxia and shock [4,33]. Further, an increase in ISS is associated with an increase in the incidence of coagulopathy that is not related to the amount of fluid administered [37].

Altered central thermoregulation, decreased heat production because of tissue hypoperfusion, exposure to low ambient temperature, and the infusion of inadequately warmed resuscitation fluids means that patients who have major trauma are often hypothermic [38]. A decrease in body temperature below 34°C is known to slow enzyme reactions of the clotting system [39], impairing thrombin generation and the formation of platelet plugs and fibrin clots while increasing clot lysis [40,41]. Acidosis (pH <7.1) also exerts an inhibitory effect on clotting enzymes and may exacerbate coagulopathy [33].

An additional contributing factor to coagulopathy is the often marked dilution of clotting factors and platelets caused by infusion of large volumes of resuscitative crystalloid and colloid fluids and the transfusion of RBC units

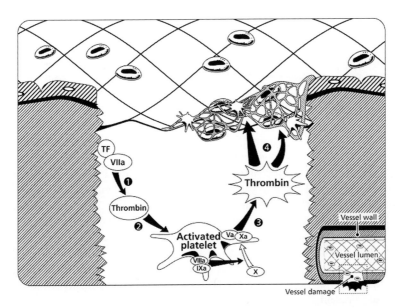

Fig. 1. Overview of hemostasis and the coagulation process [36,37]. On vessel wall injury, tissue factor (TF) is exposed to circulating endogenous factor VII/VIIa, leading to the TF/VIIa complex, which initiates coagulation (1). A limited amount of thrombin activates factors V, VIII, and platelets (2). Activation of factor X leads to the formation of the prothrombinase complex Xa/Va, which subsequently generates large amounts of thrombin (3). This thrombin burst induces the generation of a hemostatic plug that prevents further blood loss (4).

devoid of appreciable levels of platelets and essential coagulation factors. Although RBC transfusion is life saving in trauma patients who have hemorrhagic shock, in cases in which massive transfusion is required (in excess of 10 units of RBC), coagulopathy and thrombocytopenia are common [30,32,42].

Overcoming coagulopathy

In theory, blood-component therapy offers scope for the optimal use of RBCs, platelets, plasma, and fibrinogen or cryoprecipitate in accord with the patient's needs [43,44]. There are no universally accepted guidelines as to how best to use these blood components to restore normal coagulation, however. Instead recommendations are based on personal experience or experts' opinions rather than on evidence from randomized controlled trials [32]. In practice, a stepwise approach to replacement therapy is used. The first step involves empiric prophylactic administration of fresh frozen plasma (FFP) after a certain number of units of RBCs have been transfused [45]. There is no consensus on the optimal ratio of FFP to RBCs or of platelets to RBCs and no conclusive evidence that such practices prevent the development of coagulopathy or improve bleeding [32].

The second step is to use component therapies when there is clinical evidence of coagulopathy, for example when there is microvascular diffuse bleeding or when laboratory evidence suggests coagulopathy [44]. When a patient has evident microvascular bleeding, a hematocrit of 21% to 24%, a prothrombin time (PT) or an activated partial thromboplastin time (aPTT) more than 1.5 times normal, thrombocytopenia with a platelet count of under $50 \times 10^9/L$, or fibrinogen concentration less than 1 g/L, coagulopathy can be considered. In such cases, these values may act as trigger points for blood component treatment (Fig. 2) [46]. Although there are guidelines from the American Society of Anesthesiologists (ASA) for replacement therapy in patients who have coagulopathy (Table 1) [32], reliance on laboratory markers and measures of coagulopathy has major shortcomings in trauma. Often, results of laboratory tests are provided too late (30–60 minutes after sampling) to be of use. The hemostatic status of a trauma patient can be subject to precipitous change, and the practice of rewarming and buffering samples for assay may lead to a failure to detect or an underestimate of hypothermia- or acidosis-related coagulopathies [32]. Attempts should therefore be made to correct acidosis and hypothermia if clinically present.

A further limitation of component replacement therapy is that in preparation and storage of platelets and FFP significant losses can occur, such that even transfusion of RBCs, FFP, and platelets in a 1:1:1 ratio does not necessarily reconstitute coagulation [32]. During preparation of FFP, levels of coagulation factors are diluted by approximately 15% and further

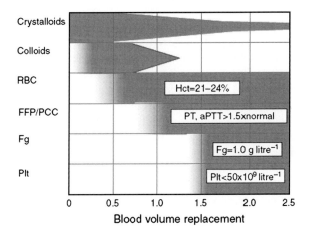

Fig. 2. Fluid and blood component treatment in major bleeding; parameters and trigger points for transfusion of components and concentrates. Fg, fibrinogen; Hct, hematocrit; PCC, prothrombin complex concentrate; Plt, platelets. (*Adapted from* Erber WN. Massive blood transfusion in the elective surgical setting. Transfus Apheresis Sci 2002;27:83–92; with permission from European Society of Haemapheresis.)

losses are believed to occur during freezing and thawing [47]. Massive transfusion of blood products is associated with worsened clinical outcome, however, and more than 50% of patients who receive massive transfusion after trauma do not survive their hospital stay [48,49]. In trauma there is a known dose relationship between high RBC transfusion and the likelihood of multiple organ failure (MOF) requiring intensive care unit stay [48–50]. Although the mechanism of increased organ damage attributable to RBC transfusion has not been firmly established, it is believed that during storage bioreactive lipids are generated by RBCs, which may contribute to heightened systemic inflammatory responses [48]. Artificial oxygen carriers are a novel class of colloids capable of transporting and off-loading oxygen to tissues. These substances are in development but are not yet approved by health authorities in the Western world [51].

Table 1
The ASA 1996 guidelines for replacement therapy in patients who have coagulopathy

Coagulation parameter	Recommended replacement therapy
PT >1.5 times normal	FFP, prothrombin complex concentrate
aPTT >1.5 times normal	FFP
Fibrinogen <1.0 g/L	Fibrinogen concentrate, cryoprecipitate
Platelets <50 × 10^9/L	Platelets

From Spahn DR, Rossaint R. Coagulopathy and blood component transfusion in trauma. Br J Anaesth 2005;95:130–9; with permission.

Adjunctive use of recombinant activated factor VIIa

As a third step (Fig. 3), a novel approach to the management of coagulopathic bleeding may be considered: adjunctive use of rFVIIa, a blood clotting factor shown to provide effective hemostasis in a range of bleeding conditions characterized by impaired thrombin generation and life-threatening bleeding [52,53]. rFVIIa is widely used in the management of bleeding in hemophilia patients with inhibitors and, while not currently indicated for use in the management of trauma bleeding, has demonstrated efficacy in case series and most recently in randomized controlled studies in patients who have multiple trauma [54–56].

rFVIIa has a mode of action founded on physiologic coagulation processes [37,57]. At pharmacologic doses, rFVIIa binds to the surface of locally activated platelets, activating factor X, which results in enhanced localized thrombin generation and formation of a stable fibrin clot at the site of vascular injury.

Recently, the results of two randomized controlled studies of rFVIIa for control of bleeding in patients who had severe trauma (blunt and penetrating injury) were published [56]. In these studies, the primary endpoint was number of RBC units transfused during the first 48 hours after first dose of trial product. Patients had severe traumatic bleeding, defined as the need for transfusion of six units of RBCs within 4 hours of admission, and on completion of the eighth unit of RBC they received three injections of rFVIIa (200 μg/kg followed by 100 μg/kg and 100 μg/kg 1 and 3 hours later, respectively) or placebo, in addition to local standard blood component and surgical treatment for hemorrhage.

When patients who died within the first 48 hours were excluded from the analyses (an a priori decision), the reduction in RBC requirement among patients who had blunt injuries was significant (an estimated reduction of 2.6 total RBC units per patient [$P = .02$]). In these blunt trauma patients, the need for massive transfusion—defined here as need for more than 20 units RBCs—was significantly reduced by rFVIIa treatment from 33% to 14% ($P = .03$), a relative risk reduction of 56% (Fig. 4) [56]. There was a significant treatment-related reduction in acute respiratory distress syndrome (ARDS) at 30 days in blunt trauma patients, from 16% (placebo) to 4% (rFVIIa) ($P = .03$). Despite similar trends toward improved bleeding control and outcome in patients who had penetrating trauma, no statistically significant benefits of therapy were observed in these patients [56]. In both studies, adverse event rates between placebo- and rFVIIa-treated groups were similar, with no differences in the rate of thromboembolic events (Table 2). The issue of possible thromboembolic events associated with rFVIIa use requires further investigation in large-scale randomized clinical studies, because evidence to date (reports to the Food and Drug Administration) shows that analysis of the relationship between rFVIIa and adverse events is often hindered by concomitant medications and preexisting medical conditions and confounded by indication [58].

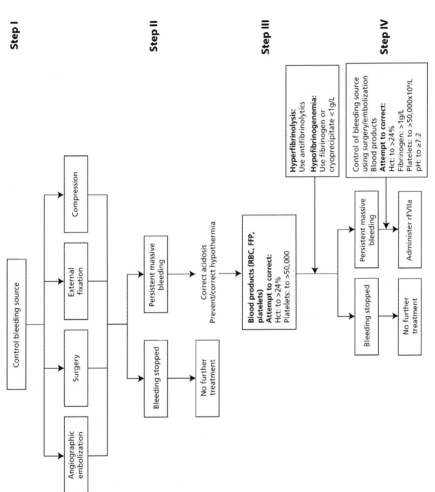

Fig. 3. Stepwise management of traumatic bleeding and an algorithm for the use of rFVIIa. Hct, hematocrit.

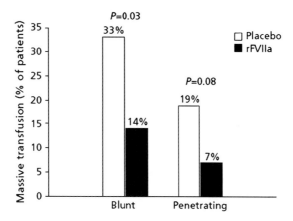

Fig. 4. Massive transfusion. Percentages of patients alive at 48 hours receiving more than 12 units of RBCs within 48 hours of the first dose, which equals >20 units of RBCs (inclusive of 8 predose units). (*From* Boffard KD, Riou B, Warren B, et al for the NovoSeven Trauma Study Group. Recombinant factor VIIa as adjunctive therapy for bleeding control in severely injured trauma patients: two parallel randomized, placebo-controlled, double-blind clinical trials. J Trauma 2005;59:8–15; with permission.)

These first controlled studies of rFVIIa in trauma suggest a potential place for rFVIIa in the management of trauma patients who have nonsurgical coagulopathic bleeding. The reductions in RBC requirements noted in these studies can be expected to translate into improvements in patients' long-term clinical outcome [48–50,59].

Summary

There is an urgent need for improved strategies to control bleeding in patients who have major trauma in which hemorrhage is a major preventable cause of death. Wider use of angiographic embolization, better understanding of trauma-related coagulopathy, and the publication of randomized controlled studies showing efficacy for the hemostatic agent rFVIIa are providing clinicians with data on new adjunctive tools with which to control the coagulopathic diffuse bleeding that often occurs in trauma despite best efforts to control bleeding through traditional means.

Acknowledgments

The authors acknowledge Winnie McFazdean of PAREXEL MMS for medical writing services in the preparation of this manuscript, which were financially supported by Novo Nordisk.

Table 2
Adverse events and clinical outcomes

	Blunt trauma			Penetrating trauma		
	Placebo (n = 74)	rFVIIa (n = 69)	P value	Placebo (n = 64)	RFVIIa (n = 70)	P value
Serious adverse events						
Patients with events	49 (66%)	44 (64%)	—	36 (56%)	36 (51%)	—
Number of events	109	91	—	76	57	—
Thromboembolic adverse events						
Patients with events	3 (4%)	2 (3%)	—	3 (5%)	4 (6%)	—
Number of events	3	2	—	3	4	—
48-hour mortality	13 (18%)	13 (19%)	1.00	10 (16%)	12 (17%)	1.00
30-day mortality	22 (30%)	17 (25%)	0.58	18 (28%)	17 (24%)	0.69
Patients who have critical complications within 30 days						
ARDS	12 (16%)	3 (4%)	0.03	5 (8%)	4 (6%)	0.74
MOF	9 (12%)	5 (7%)	0.41	7 (11%)	2 (3%)	0.09
Patients who have ARDS, MOF or death	31 (42%)	20 (29%)	0.16	22 (34%)	20 (29%)	0.57
Ventilator-free days[a] (median and range)	13 (0–29)	17 (0–29)	0.43	20 (0–29)	25 (0–29)	0.21
ICU-free days[a] (median and range)	8 (0–29)	12 (0–29)	0.31	18 (0–29)	23 (0–29)	0.34

[a] Within 30 days of trial product treatment.

From Boffard KD, Riou B, Warren B, et al, for the NovoSeven Trauma Study Group. Recombinant factor VIIa as adjunctive therapy for bleeding control in severely injured trauma patients: two parallel randomized, placebo-controlled, double-blind clinical trials. J Trauma 2005;59:8–15; with permission.

References

[1] Peden M, McGee K, Sharma G. The injury chart book: a graphical overview of the global burden of injuries. Geneva (Switzerland): World Health Organization; 2002.

[2] Murray CJ, Lopez AD. Mortality by cause for eight regions of the world: global burden of disease study. Lancet 1997;349(9061):1269–76.

[3] Holcomb JB. Methods for improved hemorrhage control. Crit Care 2004;8(Suppl 2):S57–60.

[4] Hoyt DB. A clinical review of bleeding dilemmas in trauma. Semin Hematol 2004;41 (1 Suppl 1):40–3.

[5] Sauaia A, Moore FA, Moore EE, et al. Epidemiology of trauma deaths: a reassessment. J Trauma 1995;38(2):185–93.

[6] Ertel W, Eid K, Keel M, et al. Therapeutic strategies and outcome of polytraumatized patients with pelvic injuries. A six year experience. Eur J Trauma 2000;26:278–86.

[7] Stahel PF, Heyde CE, Ertel W. Current concepts of polytrauma management. Eur J Trauma 2005;31:200–11.

[8] Keel M, Labler L, Trentz O. "Damage Control" in severely injured patients. Why, when and how? Eur J Trauma 2005;31:212–21.

[9] Parr MJA, Alabdi T. Damage control surgery and intensive care. Injury 2004;35(7):713–22.

[10] Giannoudis PV, Pape HC. Damage control orthopaedics in unstable pelvic ring injuries. Injury 2004;35(7):671–7.

[11] Rotondo MF, Bard MR. Damage control surgery for thoracic injuries. Injury 2004;35(7): 649–54.

[12] Hildebrand F, Giannoudis P, Krettek C, et al. Damage control: extremities. Injury 2004; 35(7):678–89.

[13] MacLeod JB, Lynn M, McKenney MG, et al. Early coagulopathy predicts mortality in trauma. J Trauma 2003;55(1):39–44.

[14] Panetta T, Sclafani SJ, Goldstein AS, et al. Percutaneous transcatheter embolization for massive bleeding from pelvic fractures. J Trauma 1985;25(11):1021–9.

[15] Velmahos GC, Chahwan S, Falabella A, et al. Angiographic embolization for intraperitoneal and retroperitoneal injuries. World J Surg 2000;24(5):539–45.

[16] Velmahos GC, Toutouzas KG, Vassiliu P, et al. A prospective study on the safety and efficacy of angiographic embolization for pelvic and visceral injuries. J Trauma 2002;53(2):303–8.

[17] Eastridge BJ, Starr A, Minei JP, et al. The importance of fracture pattern in guiding therapeutic decision-making in patients with hemorrhagic shock and pelvic ring disruptions. J Trauma 2002;53(3):446–50.

[18] Hagiwara A, Yukioka T, Ohta S, et al. Nonsurgical management of patients with blunt splenic injury: efficacy of transcatheter arterial embolization. Am J Roentgenol 1996; 167(1):159–66.

[19] Haan J, Scott J, Boyd-Kranis RL, et al. Admission angiography for blunt splenic injury: advantages and pitfalls. J Trauma 2001;51(6):1161–5.

[20] Shanmuganathan K, Mirvis SE, Boyd-Kranis R, et al. Nonsurgical management of blunt splenic injury: use of CT criteria to select patients for splenic arteriography and potential endovascular therapy. Radiology 2000;217(1):75–82.

[21] Scalea TM, Burgess AR. Pelvic fracture. In: Mattox KL, Feliciano DV, Moore EE, editors. Trauma. New York: McGraw-Hill; 2000. p. 823–6.

[22] Fangio P, Asehnoune K, Edouard A, et al. Early embolization and vasopressor administration for management of life-threatening hemorrhage from pelvic fracture. J Trauma 2005; 58(5):978–84.

[23] Hagiwara A, Murata A, Matsuda T, et al. The usefulness of transcatheter arterial embolization for patients with blunt polytrauma showing transient response to fluid resuscitation. J Trauma 2004;57(2):271–6.

[24] Heetveld MJ, Harris I, Schlaphoff G, et al. Guidelines for the management of haemodynamically unstable pelvic fracture patients. ANZ J Surg 2004;74(7):520–9.

[25] Agolini SF, Shah K, Jaffe J, et al. Arterial embolization is a rapid and effective technique for controlling pelvic fracture hemorrhage. J Trauma 1997;43(3):395–9.
[26] Sarin EL, Moore JB, Moore EE, et al. Pelvic fracture pattern does not always predict the need for urgent embolization. J Trauma 2005;58(5):973–7.
[27] Miller PR, Moore PS, Mansell E, et al. External fixation or arteriogram in bleeding pelvic fracture: initial therapy guided by markers of arterial hemorrhage. J Trauma 2003;54(3): 437–43.
[28] Perez JV, Hughes TM, Bowers K. Angiographic embolisation in pelvic fracture. Injury 1998; 29(3):187–91.
[29] Yasumura K, Ikegami K, Kamohara T, et al. High incidence of ischemic necrosis of the gluteal muscle after transcatheter angiographic embolization for severe pelvic fracture. J Trauma 2005;58(5):985–90.
[30] Shafi S, Kauder DR. Fluid resuscitation and blood replacement in patients with polytrauma. Clin Orthop Rel Res 2004;422:37–42.
[31] Bilkovski RN, Rivers EP, Horst HM. Targeted resuscitation strategies after injury. Curr Opin Crit Care 2004;10(6):529–38.
[32] Spahn DR, Rossaint R. Coagulopathy and blood component transfusion in trauma. Br J Anaesth 2005;95(2):130–9.
[33] Lynn M, Jeroukhimov I, Klein Y, et al. Updates in the management of severe coagulopathy in trauma patients. Intensive Care Med 2002;28(Suppl 2):S241–7.
[34] Cosgriff N, Moore EE, Sauia A, et al. Predicting life-threatening coagulopathy in the massively transfused trauma patient. Hypothermia and acidosis revisited. J Trauma 1997;42(5): 857–61.
[35] Bombeli T, Spahn DR. Updates on perioperative coagulation: physiology and management of thromboembolism and hemorrhage. Br J Anaesth 2004;93(2):275–87.
[36] Monroe DM, Hoffman M. What does it take to make the perfect clot? Arterioscler Thromb Vasc Biol 2006;26(1):41–8.
[37] Monroe DM, Hoffman M, Oliver JA, et al. A possible mechanism of action of activated factor VII independent of tissue factor. Blood Coagul Fibrinolysis 1998;9(1):S15–20.
[38] Brohi K, Singh J, Heron M, et al. Acute traumatic coagulopathy. J Trauma 2003;54(6): 1127–30.
[39] Krause KR, Howells GA, Buhs CL, et al. Hypothermia-induced coagulopathy during hemorrhagic shock. Am Surg 2000;66(4):348–54.
[40] Wolberg AS, Meng ZG, Monroe DM III, et al. A systematic evaluation of the effect of temperature on coagulation enzyme activity and platelet function. J Trauma 2004;56(6):1221–8.
[41] Meng ZH, Wolberg AS, Monroe DM III, et al. The effect of temperature and pH on the activity of factor VIIa in hypothermic and acidotic patients. J Trauma 2003;55(5):886–91.
[42] Hardy JF, Samama M. Massive transfusion and coagulopathy. Transfusion Alternatives in Transfusion Medicine 2003;4(3):199–210.
[43] Council of Europe Publishing. Guide to the preparation, use and quality assurance of blood components. 10th edition. Strasburg (France): Council of Europe Publishing; 2004.
[44] Practice guidelines for blood component therapy: a report by the American Society of Anesthesiologists Task Force on blood component therapy. Anesthesiology 1996;84(3):732–47.
[45] Hiippala S. Replacement of massive blood loss. Vox Sang 1998;74(Suppl 2):399–407.
[46] Erber WN. Massive blood transfusion in the elective surgery setting. Transfus Apheresis Sci 2002;27(1):83–92.
[47] Chowdhury P, Saaman AG, Paulus U, et al. Efficacy of standard dose and 30 ml/kg fresh frozen plasma in correcting laboratory parameters of haemostasis in critically ill patients. Br J Haematol 2004;125(1):69–73.
[48] Moore FA, Moore EE, Sauaia A. Blood transfusion. An independent risk factor for postinjury multiple organ failure. Arch Surg 1997;132(6):620–4.
[49] Vaslef SN, Knudsen NW, Neligan PJ, et al. Massive transfusion exceeding 50 units of blood products in trauma patients. J Trauma 2002;53(2):291–5.

[50] Malone DL, Dunne J, Tracy JK, et al. Blood transfusion, independent of shock severity, is associated with worse outcome in trauma. J Trauma 2003;54(5):898–905.
[51] Spahn DR, Kocian R. Artificial O_2 carriers: status in 2005. Curr Pharm Des 2005;11(31): 4099–114.
[52] Jurlander B, Thim L, Klausen NK, et al. Recombinant activated factor VII (rFVIIa): characterization, manufacturing, and clinical development. Semin Thromb Hemost 2001; 27(4):373–83.
[53] Levi M, Peters M, Buller HR. Efficacy and safety of recombinant factor VIIa for treatment of severe bleeding: a systematic review. Crit Care Med 2005;33(4):883–90.
[54] Dutton RP, McCunn M, Hyder M, et al. Factor VIIa for correction of traumatic coagulopathy. J Trauma 2004;57(4):709–18.
[55] Martinowitz U, Michaelson M. The Israeli Multidisciplinary rFVIIa Task Force. Guidelines for the use of recombinant activated factor VII (rFVIIa) in uncontrolled bleeding: a report by the Israeli Multidisciplinary rFVIIa Task Force. J Thromb Haemost 2005;3(4):640–8.
[56] Boffard KD, Riou B, Warren B, et al, for the NovoSeven® Trauma Study Group. Recombinant factor VIIa as adjunctive therapy for bleeding control in severely injured trauma patients: two parallel randomized, placebo-controlled, double-blind clinical trials. J Trauma 2005;59(1):8–15.
[57] Hoffman M, Monroe DM, Roberts HR. Activated factor VII activates factors IX and X on the surface of activated platelets: thoughts on the mechanism of action of high-dose activated factor VII. Blood Coagul Fibrinolysis 1998;9(1):S61–5.
[58] O'Connell KA, Wood JJ, Wise RP, et al. Thromboembolic adverse events after use of recombinant human coagulation factor VIIa. JAMA 2006;295(3):293–8.
[59] Claridge JA, Sawyer RG, Schulman AM, et al. Blood transfusions correlate with infections in trauma patients in a dose-dependent manner. Am Surg 2002;68(7):566–72.

ELSEVIER
SAUNDERS

Anesthesiology Clin
25 (2007) 49–63

ANESTHESIOLOGY
CLINICS

Trauma and Aggressive Homeostasis Management

Dimitry Baranov, MD*, Patrick Neligan, MA, MD

*Department of Anesthesiology and Critical Care, Hospital of University of Pennsylvania,
3400 Spruce Street, Philadelphia, PA 19104, USA*

Homeostasis refers to the capacity of the human body to maintain a stable, constant state by detecting and controlling deviations from the normal range in vital functions. Patients who undergo tissue injury, such as trauma or surgery, undergo a well-understood, reproducible, metabolic, and neuroendocrine stress response. The ability of the body to deal with stress is known as physiologic reserve, the excess capacity in organ systems that deals with injury and allows the body to restore homeostasis. The cardiovascular system, lungs, kidneys, and liver have enormous functional reserve. Aging and chronic illness deplete physiologic reserve. Critical illness is a state in which physiologic reserve is inadequate to maintain life, and exogenous organ support is required.

In this article, the authors discuss three issues concerning homeostasis in the acute care of trauma patients that are related directly to the stress response: hyperglycemia, lactic acidosis, and hypothermia. Recently, there has been a resurgence of interest in investigating the effects of aggressive thermal and glucose concentration and volume resuscitation on outcomes in critically ill and trauma patients. Significant reason exists to question the "conventional wisdom" relating to current approaches to restoring homeostasis in this patient population.

Hyperglycemia and trauma

Trauma is associated with changes in metabolism and neurohormonal function, often referred to as the "stress" response. Key to this response is the presence of white cells in the damaged tissues. These cells phagocytose cellular debris, secrete growth factors, and catalyze the synthesis of collagen.

---

* Corresponding author.
E-mail address: baranovd@uphs.upenn.edu (D. Baranov).

0889-8537/07/$ - see front matter © 2007 Elsevier Inc. All rights reserved.
doi:10.1016/j.atc.2006.11.003
anesthesiology.theclinics.com

As part of this response, blood glucose levels increase dramatically because of enhanced glycogenolysis and gluconeogenesis. This homeostatic mechanism mobilizes substrate, principally from the liver and skeletal muscle, to restore function, fight infection, and repair damaged tissue. White cells are obligate glucose users. Hyperglycemia is facilitated by a dramatic increase in the secretion of cortisol, growth hormone, epinephrine, and glucagon. Epinephrine induces glycogenolysis, lipolysis, and increased lactate production, independent of cellular redox state [1]. This process has been termed "aerobic glycolysis." Simultaneous increases in insulin production lead to increased peripheral glucose uptake [2]. The apparent ceiling glycemic concentration above which hyperglycemia is associated with adverse outcomes has lead to an interest in the benefits of "tight glycemic control" [3,4].

It is important to differentiate association and causality. Currently, no data exist to implicate stress hyperglycemia and adverse outcomes in trauma; however, substantial data are available in other clinical and laboratory conditions [5–7]. Hyperglycemia can lead to dehydration by inducing diuresis. Hyperglycemia can also induce immune dysfunction by promoting inflammation caused by induced abnormalities of white cell function [8,9]. These include granulocyte adhesion, chemotaxis, phagocytosis, respiratory burst and superoxide formation, and intracellular killing [7]. Hyperglycemia negatively affects wound healing [10]. A limitation of these claims is that the studies were performed in diabetic patients, not those with stress hyperglycemia; immune suppression may result from the disease, one of absolute or relative insulin deficiency, rather than the glucose.

Clinical data suggest that hyperglycemia and poorly controlled diabetes result in worse outcomes from myocardial ischemia and stroke [5,11–13]. In trauma patients, a series of studies have associated the magnitude of hyperglycemia with adverse outcomes [13–20]. A question that arises is whether hyperglycemia results in poorer outcomes or whether hyperglycemia is a marker of severity of illness, analogous to hypoalbuminemia [21].

Hyperglycemia is associated with worsened outcomes in patients with brain injury [22]. However, this may be consequent of the magnitude of the stress response, rather than a result of glucose itself [23]. Animal models of stroke demonstrated that hyperglycemia in the presence of cerebral ischemia may be detrimental [24]. Hyperglycemia may worsen prognosis as a result of increased brain tissue acidosis, accumulation of extracellular glutamate, increased blood brain barrier permeability, and increased formation of cerebral edema. Hyperglycemia leads to localized tissues acidosis [25], and this in turn may increase the risk of ischemia in the penumbra [26]. Consequently, clinicians have used observational data, animal studies [24], and human studies in different fields [27,28] to justify tight glycemic control in this patient population.

In view of the association between adverse outcomes and hyperglycemia, it has been proposed that aggressive control of glucose plasma concentration may improve outcomes. Analogously, intensive insulin therapy may be used to achieve glycemic control. Insulin has significant anti-inflammatory properties and antioxidant activity, and reduces the quantity of circulating cytokines [29].

Obese patients who have insulin-resistant type 2 diabetics have larger infarcts than nondiabetics. In a rat model of myocardial ischemia, the introduction of insulin into the reperfusion fluid reduced infarct size by 50% [30]. A similar effect was seen in humans given insulin, Tissue Plasminogen Activator, and heparin [31].

Does intensive insulin therapy improve outcomes in perioperative and critically ill patients? Zerr, Furnari and colleagues [32–34] demonstrated that meticulous control of blood glucose significantly reduces the incidence of deep sternal wound infections and perioperative mortality in diabetic patients undergoing cardiac surgery.

Insulin appears to be cardioprotective in the presence of ischemia [30,35]. Insulin therapy in perioperative, and, in particular, cardiothoracic surgical patients, was associated with a significant reduction in the risk of death [27]. Enthusiasm for insulin therapy, rather than glycemic control, must be tempered by the knowledge that increased insulin administration is associated positively with death in the ICU, regardless of the prevailing blood glucose level [36]. Additionally, it remains unclear whether these data may be applicable in other clinical situations.

In one prospective, randomized, unblinded clinical trial of 1548 patients admitted to the surgical ICU, patients were randomized into two groups. The conventional therapy group received an insulin drip adjusted to maintain a blood glucose of 180 to 200 mg/dL [37]. The second group received "intensive insulin therapy": an insulin drip was started if blood glucose exceeded 100 mg/dL, and the level was adjusted to maintain blood glucose between 80 and 100 mg/dL. Overall, intensive insulin therapy resulted in an absolute risk reduction of death of 3.4%. Subgroup analysis suggested that this mortality difference accrued principally to patients who were critically ill, rather than those who underwent a standard perioperative stress response. Given the small number of trauma patients, it is unlikely that this study is applicable to that patient population. It was also concluded that glycemic control was more important than insulin dose [37,38]. Indeed, increasing the insulin dose was related to an increased incidence of renal failure in this study [37]. Finney and colleagues [36] showed that increased insulin administration is positively associated with death in the ICU, regardless of the prevailing blood glucose level.

A single-center cohort study of intensive insulin therapy versus recent historic controls found a significant reduction in hospital mortality, ICU length of stay, and blood transfusion [39].

Van Den Berght's group [40] followed their initial report with a study of intensive insulin therapy in the medical ICU. Twelve hundred patients were enrolled in the study. Mortality outcomes were not statistically different (37.3% in the intensive insulin therapy group versus 40.0% in the conventional therapy group ($P = .33$). Subgroup analysis suggested that patients who stayed in the ICU for more than 3 days benefited from insulin therapy, although it is difficult to interpret the usefulness of these data.

The issue of hypoglycemia cannot be ignored. A German multicenter study of intensive insulin therapy in patients who had severe sepsis was stopped early because of a significant excess risk of severe hypoglycemia without any evidence of improved survival [41,42]. The brain depends on glucose as its main source of energy; thus, a significant blood-to-brain-glucose gradient is required. Vespa and colleagues [43] have shown that a cerebral microdialysis glucose level of 0.2 mmol/L or less during intensive glucose control is an independent predictor of bad outcome in a traumatic brain injury (TBI). Hence, care must be taken to avoid hypoglycemia in patients who have TBI receiving intravenous insulin. The margin between beneficial and detrimental effects appears to be narrow.

In summary, current data do not support intensive insulin therapy in victims of trauma. Although many neuroscientists have translated data from animal and clinical studies of stroke patients to TBI, tight glycemic control has not been studied prospectively in this patient population.

Lactate, tissue acidosis, and trauma

The objective of volume replacement during trauma resuscitation is to restore tissue perfusion. Unfortunately, conventional clinical and laboratory signs, such as heart rate, blood pressure, and hemoglobin, may be misleading in trauma patients [44].

As early as the 1980s, it was observed that hypothermia, coagulopathy, and acidosis constituted a "triad of death" in trauma victims [45]. The mechanism of acidosis is presumed to be cellular oxygen debt, secondary to hypoperfusion or hypoxia. The anion implicated in this acidosis is lactate. Acidosis has a negative inotropic effect, induces vasoplegia, shifts the oxyhemoglobin dissociation curve rightwards, and is thought to reduce the effectiveness of vasopressors. In addition, acidosis may reduce splanchnic perfusion, including glomerular filtration rate.

The ability to measure serum lactate was not available universally until recently, and a surrogate, the base deficit [46], has be used for 2 decades. Care should be taken using this tool, and inferences about its validity should be placed in the context of quantitative acid base chemistry [47–50]. In the setting of acute trauma, there may be multiple acidifying and alkalinizing processes occurring simultaneously, depending on the volume and nature of intravenous fluids [51]. A "normal" base deficit or excess may hide potentially dangerous acid-base disturbances [51]. Base deficit does not reflect lactate reliably in the emergency setting [49,52,53].

Lactic acidosis upon admission to the emergency room is a marker of the severity of illness. The magnitude of acidosis and the degree of elevation of serum lactate correlate well with patient outcomes [45,54,55]. The speed of clearance of lactate from the circulation is also a known prognostic indicator [55–58], which has led to an era of hyperaggresive volume resuscitation to "wash out lactate," under the assumption that serum lactate is a marker of tissue hypoperfusion. In the study by McNelis [57], lactate clearance was significantly lower in nonsurvivors. However, there was no difference in oxygen delivery and consumption between survivors and nonsurvivors [57], indicating that although admission lactate and lactate clearance may be independent predictors of mortality, the mechanism of hyperlactemia may not necessarily be hypoperfusion. In addition, lactate itself may be harmless [1,59,60]. Lactate is an important intermediate in the process of wound healing and repair. Lactate enhances collagen production and deposition, and angiogenesis [61]. Oxygen levels have little impact on wound lactate [1].

Emerging evidence indicates that lactic acidosis in trauma and critical illness may not be caused by hypoxemia, but by epinephrine-driven aerobic glycolysis [60,62], which results from cyclic AMP medicated Na^+-$K+$ ATPase activity driven by beta-adrenoceptor activation [63]. Administration of beta-adrenergic agents increases tissue lactate levels; administration of anti-adrenergic agents reduces tissue lactate levels [60].

It is widely believed that hyperglycemia predisposes to ischemia brain damage consequent of increased anaerobic glycolysis, lactate production, and tissue acidosis [64]. However, the brain is glucose-dependent and glycolysis supplies energy for metabolism during hypoxemia. In addition, lactate may be a source of energy during the postischemia state. Thus, we have the "glucose paradox of cerebral ischemia," in which increased energy delivery appears to be associated with worsened outcomes [65].

Elevated blood glucose and lactate are associated with stress; stress is associated with increase blood corticosteroid levels. An alternative hypothesis suggests that elevated serum cortisol may be related to brain injury [65]. A number of observations in animal studies have indicated that the timing of hyperglycemia before and after ischemic brain injuries significantly changes outcomes. The application of corticosteroid inhibitors reduced the severity of brain injuries, but the application of steroid increased the severity [65].

In summary, in trauma and critical illness, increased lactate levels may result from a medley of processes unrelated to oxygen delivery and hypoxemia. The assumption that elevated serum lactate is a marker of tissue hypoperfusion, rather than a marker of inflammation, has led to an approach to resuscitation (aggressive fluid administration until lactate clears) that may result in significant hypervolemia. Indeed, in the setting of acute severe trauma, elevated serum lactate represents a homeostatic mechanism, and prolonged lactate clearance represents prolonged hyperadrenergic activity.

Hypothermia and trauma

Mild to moderate hypothermia is found routinely on admission in severe trauma victims, resulting from environmental and iatrogenic factors:

exposure, large volumes of unwarmed resuscitative fluids and blood products, anesthetic agents, or intoxication with alcohol or drugs. In addition, the patient's capacity to produce heat internally may be limited severely because of impairment of the thermoregulatory mechanisms and reduced oxygen delivery to tissues in hemorrhagic shock (HS).

Accidental hypothermia, even in uninjured victims, is a significant risk factor for mortality [66]. Multiple clinical retrospective studies have demonstrated an association between exposure hypothermia and a poor outcome in trauma. Accordingly, the American College of Surgeons Advanced Trauma Life Support Program recommends prevention, prompt detection, and treatment of hypothermia in trauma patients, based on the hypothesis that, because hypothermia is associated with a higher risk of mortality in trauma patients, prevention of hypothermia, or rewarming, will lead to improved outcomes. This conclusion may be derived from epidemiology rather than pathophysiology.

Historically, induced hypothermia (IH) has been used to protect organs, in particular the brain, in cardiac, neuro-, and transplant surgery. IH has been used, on and off, as a therapeutic option in the management of TBI since it was first proposed more than 50 years ago [67]. More recently, mild to moderate IH has been shown to have a significant neuroprotective effect in multiple laboratory and clinical models of ischemic and TBI. Resuscitated victims of cardiac arrest have been shown to benefit greatly from IH [68–70]. Numerous laboratory studies have also indicated that induced mild hypothermia improves survival in laboratory animals after traumatic HS.

These data seem to conflict with a well-established belief that hypothermia has a deleterious impact on the morbidity and mortality of major trauma victims. Does hypothermia independently increase patient risk in HS and trauma, or is it a consequence of these injuries? Do hypothermic trauma patients need to be rewarmed actively, or is there some beneficial protective/therapeutic effect in allowing, and even inducing, a certain degree of hypothermia in some of these patients? To resolve these conflicts, the reader must understand the differences in the pathophysiology of accidental and other types of IH in trauma victims.

Hypothermia can be accidental or induced. Typically, major trauma is associated with accidental hypothermia, which is characteristically uncontrolled. Conversely, IH is used for preventive or therapeutic purposes, and is well-controlled and monitored. IH can be protective–preservative (pre- and intra-insult) or resuscitative–therapeutic (postinsult) [71]. For example, protective hypothermia has been used universally in cardiac surgery for brain protection. The use of therapeutic hypothermia as an adjunct to resuscitation was first proposed in the 1950s, but has only recently been validated in resuscitated victims of out-of-hospital cardiac arrest [72,73].

Hypothermia is often classified according to arbitrary chosen ranges in body temperature as mild (34–36°C), moderate (30–33°C), or deep hypothermia (<30°C). Therapeutic IH is characteristically mild to moderate.

Poor outcomes in major trauma victims usually are associated with deeper degrees of accidental hypothermia. Additionally, HS and isolated TBI victims are two separate entities with very different pathophysiologies; this requires a separate discussion about the role of hypothermia in HS and TBI patients.

Hypothermia in hemorrhagic shock

The successful use of hypothermia for organ and brain protection against hypoperfusion–ischemic injuries in cardiac surgery and organ transplantation led to interest in the use of therapeutic hypothermia for HS victims [74]. HS has been implicated in ischemic injury of vital organs caused by hypoperfusion, and is associated with high mortality rates in trauma victims. The reduction in metabolic rate associated with hypothermia potentially could alleviate the degree of ischemia in HS [75]. Additionally, mild hypothermia can reduce postischemic oxidative damage during the resuscitative phase in the treatment of HS. Mild IH during HS or during the fluid resuscitation phase improved the survival of experimental animals in the models of uncontrolled, volume-controlled [76,77], pressure-controlled [78], and prolonged HS combined with significant tissue trauma [79], compared with normothermic resuscitation. Wu and colleagues [79] created a clinically relevant animal outcome model of HS with extensive tissue damage, which included an intensive care environment similar to that found in the clinical situation. The mechanism by which hypothermia improved survival in these animals could not be determined.

Conversely, other studies found that in experimental and clinical models of HS, hypothermia adversely affected vital organs and systems. The adverse effects of hypothermia on individual vital functions may explain why hypothermia may contribute to mortality and morbidity in clinical observational studies, while being useful in laboratory experiments, where the adverse effects of hypothermia can be well controlled and monitored. For example, Mizushima [80] demonstrated that hypothermia depressed cardiac function and hepatic blood flow in an HS model. Active rewarming during resuscitation improved cardiac function and hepatic blood flow, compared with animals that were allowed to remain hypothermic. The hypothermia-rewarming group of animals had improved parameters, compared with the control group where normothermia was maintained during and after injury [80].

It has been proposed that hypothermia-induced coagulopathy is a significant contributing factor to adverse outcomes in trauma. Hypothermia, blood loss, and impaired hemostasis are strongly associated in these patients [81]. Hypothermia, below 34 to 33°C, directly impairs clotting enzyme activity [82–84] and platelet function [84,85]. It has been suggested that hypothermia and resuscitative hemodilution may have a synergistic impact on coagulation [82], which may explain the absence of an association between

IH and bleeding in laboratory experiments [86] and in clinical studies of head injury where fluid administration was restricted [87].

Another mechanism by which hypothermia may worsen outcomes in trauma patients is immunosuppression. Mild hypothermia may reduce the expression of heat shock protein, impair granulocyte recruitment, and alter cytokine balance [88,89].

A novel and promising field in hypothermia research is "suspended animation" with profound hypothermia in animal models of exsanguination cardiac arrest. Conventional resuscitation is rarely successful in trauma victims suffering cardiac arrest following exsanguinations [90]. However, it is possible that some of these patients could be saved with neurologic protection during pulselessness [91]. Safar and colleagues [92,93] in Pittsburgh have developed an approach of "buying time" for transport and resuscitative surgery during cardiac arrest, followed by delayed resuscitation, in animals. In this approach, called emergency preservation and resuscitation (EPR), profound hypothermia of the brain is achieved by rapid aortic flush with ice-called (2°C) saline, followed by delayed resuscitation with cardiopulmonary bypass. Intact survival in rapidly exsanguinated dogs was achieved with 30 minutes of EPR, induced 5 minutes after cardiac arrest. Wu and colleagues [94] have demonstrated that EPR allowed normal recovery from cardiac arrest after prolonged HS in animals unsalvageable with conventional CPR. The animals in which mild hypothermia was maintained for 36 hours after EPR had better outcomes than the animals exposed to only 12 hours of mild hypothermia after EPR. This technique has not yet been tested in clinical settings.

The magnitude of tissue injury and the degree of hypothermia are correlated strongly [95]. In earlier observational retrospective studies [96–98], investigators found that hypothermia was associated with a higher mortality, greater need for transfusion, longer hospital stay, acidosis, and higher injury severity scores. Later studies confirmed that hypothermia, independent of severity of injury and shock, was associated with increased risk of death [99–101].

Gentilello and colleagues [102] studied the effect of rapid versus standard rewarming in moderately to severely injured patients who had admission hypothermia. This study showed reduced fluid and blood product requirements, reduced length of ICU stay, and improved short-term, but not long-term, survival. This study remains the only published, prospective, randomized, controlled, clinical trial of management of hypothermia in trauma patients.

A question that needs to be asked is whether or not hypothermia per se increases mortality, or whether it is simply an indicator of depleted physiologic reserve in HS patients with greater injury severity or greater baseline risk. Retrospective clinical studies are poorly suited to address this question of causality versus association. A prospective, randomized, controlled trial is needed.

The current consensus in the literature and among traumatologists indicates that hypothermia in HS patients should be prevented and treated promptly until new evidence emerges to the contrary.

Hypothermia in traumatic brain injury

Multiple animal studies have demonstrated beneficial effects of mild to moderate IH on mortality and neurologic outcomes and brain physiologic parameters after severe TBI, generating interest in the application of this treatment modality to humans. As a result, IH following TBI has been investigated in a series of randomized, controlled trials. Clifton and colleagues [103] showed a greater complication rate in hypothermic patients, compared with normothermic patients. A multicenter Japanese study of mild hypothermia in TBI demonstrated significantly more complications, such as pneumonia and meningitis, in the hypothermic group [104]. Two meta-analyses on the use of hypothermia for the treatment of TBI came out with conflicting results: [105,106] Henderson and colleagues [105] concluded that existing evidence does not support the use of IH in an unselected group of TBI patients; McIntyre [106] found that hypothermia appears to reduce mortality and improve neurologic outcomes. Why the confusion?

The duration of hypothermia appears to be important: outcomes are improved when hypothermia is used early and for a prolonged period of time, with slower rewarming. Polderman and colleagues [107] demonstrated improved long-term survival and long-term neurologic outcome in a select group of patients who had malignant cerebral edema and intracranial hypertension refractory to other therapies, following induction of mild, prolonged hypothermia with very slow rewarming guided by intracranial pressure (ICP) monitoring.

Two randomized clinical trials [108,109] that included 396 and 215 patients, respectively, demonstrated improved outcomes in severe TBI patients with raised ICP when treated for a prolonged (5 days) period of mild hypothermia. Although these data are insufficient to recommend routine IH in TBI, the patients who appear to benefit have severe brain injury associated with raised intracranial pressure. Hypothermia should be maintained for no less than 48 hours and the rate of rewarming should be not less than 24 hours.

Summary

Trauma injury should be seen as a part of the well-defined paradigm of the stress response associated with acute depletion of physiologic reserve. Many of the observed homeostatic upsets associated with trauma can be explained as part of this process, and should not be considered pathologic. Enthusiasm for tight glycemic control in HS and TBI should be tempered by knowledge of the role of glucose in inflammation; little outcome evidence supports the use of insulin infusions in this patient population. Additionally, the use of lactate as an end point of resuscitation must be viewed with skepticism in view of emerging evidence that increased lactate in severe injury and critical illness may result from aerobic glycolysis, rather than hypoperfusion. Hypothermia and coagulopathy are strongly associated with adverse outcomes, probably a reflection of an acute depletion of physiologic reserve in patients with poorly identified predisposing factors. Data regarding therapeutic hypothermia in HS and TBI are conflicting. In the absence of better data, it is the authors' recommendation that hypothermic HS patients be kept warm or actively rewarmed on arrival in the emergency room.

References

[1] Gladden LB. Lactate metabolism: a new paradigm for the third millennium. J Physiol Online 2004;558:5–30.
[2] Lang CH, Obih JC, Bagby GJ, et al. Increased glucose uptake by intestinal mucosa and muscularis in hypermetabolic sepsis. Am J Physiol 1991;261:G287–94.
[3] Langouche L, Van den BG. Glucose metabolism and insulin therapy. Crit Care Clin 2006; 22:119–29.
[4] Gropper MA. Evidence-based management of critically ill patients: analysis and implementation. Anesth Analg 2004;99:566–72.
[5] Capes SE, Hunt D, Malmberg K, et al. Stress hyperglycaemia and increased risk of death after myocardial infarction in patients with and without diabetes: a systematic overview. Lancet 2000;355:773–8.
[6] Umpierrez GE, Isaacs SD, Bazargan N, et al. Hyperglycemia: an independent marker of in-hospital mortality in patients with undiagnosed diabetes. J Clin Endocrinol Metab 2002;87: 978–82.
[7] Montori VM, Bistrian BR, McMahon MM. Hyperglycemia in acutely ill patients. JAMA 2002;288:2167–9.
[8] Guha M, Bai W, Nadler JL, et al. Molecular mechanisms of tumor necrosis factor alpha gene expression in monocytic cells via hyperglycemia-induced oxidant stress-dependent and -independent pathways. J Biol Chem 2000;275:17728–39.
[9] Sampson MJ, Davies IR, Brown JC, et al. Monocyte and neutrophil adhesion molecule expression during acute hyperglycemia and after antioxidant treatment in type 2 diabetes and control patients. Arterioscler Thromb Vasc Biol 2002;22:1187–93.
[10] Lin LH, Hopf HW. Paradigm of the injury-repair continuum during critical illness. Crit Care Med 2003;31:S493–5.
[11] Wahab NN, Cowden EA, Pearce NJ, et al. Is blood glucose an independent predictor of mortality in acute myocardial infarction in the thrombolytic era? J Am Coll Cardiol 2002;40:1748–54.
[12] Iwakura K, Ito H, Ikushima M, et al. Association between hyperglycemia and the no-reflow phenomenon in patients with acute myocardial infarction. J Am Coll Cardiol 2003;41:1–7.
[13] O'Neill PA, Davies I, Fullerton KJ, et al. Stress hormone and blood glucose response following acute stroke in the elderly. Stroke 1991;22:842–7.
[14] Yendamuri S, Fulda GJ, Tinkoff GH. Admission hyperglycemia as a prognostic indicator in trauma. J Trauma 2003;55:33–8.
[15] Laird AM, Miller PR, Kilgo PD, et al. Relationship of early hyperglycemia to mortality in trauma patients. J Trauma 2004;56:1058–62.

[16] Sung J, Bochicchio GV, Joshi M, et al. Admission hyperglycemia is predictive of outcome in critically ill trauma patients. J Trauma 2005;59:80–3.

[17] Bochicchio GV, Sung J, Joshi M, et al. Persistent hyperglycemia is predictive of outcome in critically ill trauma patients. J Trauma 2005;58:921–4.

[18] Bochicchio GV, Salzano L, Joshi M, et al. Admission preoperative glucose is predictive of morbidity and mortality in trauma patients who require immediate operative intervention. Am.Surg 2005;71:171–4.

[19] Vogelzang M, Nijboer JM, van der Horst IC, et al. Hyperglycemia has a stronger relation with outcome in trauma patients than in other critically ill patients. J Trauma 2006;60: 873–7.

[20] Desai D, March R, Watters JM. Hyperglycemia after trauma increases with age. J Trauma 1989;29:719–23.

[21] Sung J, Bochicchio GV, Joshi M, et al. Admission serum albumin is predictive of outcome in critically ill trauma patients. Am Surg 2004;70:1099–102.

[22] Jeremitsky E, Omert LA, Dunham CM, et al. The impact of hyperglycemia on patients with severe brain injury. J Trauma 2005;58:47–50.

[23] Yang SY, Zhang S, Wang ML. Clinical significance of admission hyperglycemia and factors related to it in patients with acute severe head injury. Surg Neurol 1995;44:373–7.

[24] Garg R, Chaudhuri A, Munschauer F, et al. Hyperglycemia, insulin, and acute ischemic stroke: a mechanistic justification for a trial of insulin infusion therapy. Stroke 2006;37: 267–73.

[25] Wagner KR, Kleinholz M, de Court, et al. Hyperglycemic versus normoglycemic stroke: topography of brain metabolites, intracellular pH, and infarct size. J Cereb Blood Flow Metab 1992;12:213–22.

[26] Anderson RE, Tan WK, Martin HS, et al. Effects of glucose and PaO2 modulation on cortical intracellular acidosis, NADH redox state, and infarction in the ischemic penumbra. Stroke 1999;30(1):160–70.

[27] Van den BG, Wouters P, Weekers F, et al. Intensive insulin therapy in the surgical intensive care unit. N Engl J Med 2001;345:1359–67.

[28] Malmberg K, Ryden L, Efendic S, et al. Randomized trial of insulin-glucose infusion followed by subcutaneous insulin treatment in diabetic patients with acute myocardial infarction (DIGAMI study): effects on mortality at 1 year. J Am Coll Cardiol 1995;26: 57–65.

[29] Jeschke MG, Klein D, Bolder U, et al. Insulin attenuates the systemic inflammatory response in endotoxemic rats. Endocrinology 2004;145:4084–93.

[30] Jonassen AK, Sack MN, Mjos OD, et al. Myocardial protection by insulin at reperfusion requires early administration and is mediated via Akt and p70s6 kinase cell-survival signaling. Circ Res 2001;89:1191–8.

[31] Chaudhuri A, Janicke D, Wilson MF, et al. Anti-Inflammatory and profibrinolytic effect of insulin in acute ST-segment-elevation myocardial infarction. Circulation 2004;109:849–54.

[32] Zerr KJ, Furnary AP, Grunkemeier GL, et al. Glucose control lowers the risk of wound infection in diabetics after open heart operations. Ann Thorac Surg 1997;63:356–61.

[33] Furnari AP, Zerr KJ, Grunkemeier GL, et al. Continuous intravenous insulin infusion reduces the incidence of deep sternal wound infection in diabetic patients after cardiac surgical procedures. Ann Thorac Surg 1999;67:352–60.

[34] Furnari AP, Gao G, Grunkemeier GL, et al. Continuous insulin infusion reduces mortality in patients with diabetes undergoing coronary artery bypass grafting. J Thorac Cardiovasc Surg 2003;125:1007–21.

[35] Lazar HL, Chipkin SR, Fitzgerald CA, et al. Tight glycemic control in diabetic coronary artery bypass graft patients improves perioperative outcomes and decreases recurrent ischemic events. Circulation 2004;109:1497–502.

[36] Finney SJ, Zekveld C, Elia A, et al. Glucose control and mortality in critically ill patients. JAMA 2003;290:2041–7.

[37] Van den Berghe G, Wouters PJ, Bouillon R, et al. Outcome benefit of intensive insulin therapy in the critically ill: insulin dose versus glycemic control. Crit Care Med 2003; 31:359–66.

[38] Van den Berghe G. How does blood glucose control with insulin save lives in intensive care? J Clin Invest 2004;114:1187–95.

[39] Krinsley JS. Effect of an intensive glucose management protocol on the mortality of critically ill adult patients. Mayo Clin Proc 2004;79:992–1000.

[40] Van den Berghe G, Wilmer A, Hermans G, et al. Intensive insulin therapy in the medical ICU. N Engl J Med 2006;354:449–61.

[41] U.S. National Institutes of Health. Efficacy of volume substitution and insulin therapy in severe sepsis (VISEP trial). Available at: http://clinicaltrials.gov/show/NCT00135473. Accessed February 2007.

[42] Brunkhorst FM. Epidemiology of severe sepsis and septic shock in Germany–results from the German prevalence study. Infection 2005;33:19–20.

[43] Vespa P, Boonyaputthikul R, McArthur DL, et al. Intensive insulin therapy reduces micro-dialysis glucose values without altering glucose utilization or improving the lactate/pyruvate ratio after traumatic brain injury. Crit Care Med 2006;34:850–6.

[44] Dabrowski GP, Steinberg SM, Ferrara JJ, et al. A critical assessment of endpoints of shock resuscitation. Surg Clin North Am 2000;80:825–44.

[45] Eddy VA, Morris JA Jr, Cullinane DC. Hypothermia, coagulopathy, and acidosis. Surg Clin North Am 2000;80:845–54.

[46] Runciman WB, Skowronski GA. Pathophysiology of haemorrhagic shock. Anaesth Intensive Care 1984;12:193–205.

[47] Schlichtig R, Grogono AW, Severinghaus JW. Current status of acid-base quantitation in physiology and medicine. Anesthesiol Clin North Am 998;16:211–233.

[48] Fencl V, Leith DE. Stewart's quantitative acid-base chemistry: applications in biology and medicine. Respir Physiol 1993;91:1–16.

[49] Brill SA, Stewart TR, Brundage SI, et al. Base deficit does not predict mortality when secondary to hyperchloremic acidosis. Shock 2002;17:459–62.

[50] Stewart PA. Modern quantitative acid-base chemistry. Can J Physiol Pharmacol 1983;61: 1444–61.

[51] Fencl V, Jabor A, Kazda A, et al. Diagnosis of metabolic acid-base disturbances in critically ill patients. Am J Respir Crit Care Med 2000;162:2246–51.

[52] Kaplan LJ, Kellum JA. Initial pH, base deficit, lactate, anion gap, strong ion difference, and strong ion gap predict outcome from major vascular injury. Crit Care Med 2004;32: 1120–4.

[53] Martin MJ, FitzSullivan E, Salim A, et al. Discordance between lactate and base deficit in the surgical intensive care unit: which one do you trust? Am J Surg 2006; 191:625–30.

[54] Vitek V, Cowley RA. Blood lactate in the prognosis of various forms of shock. Ann Surg 1971;173:308–13.

[55] Husain FA, Martin MJ, Mullenix PS, et al. Serum lactate and base deficit as predictors of mortality and morbidity. Am J Surg 2003;185:485–91.

[56] Abramson D, Scalea TM, Hitchcock R, et al. Lactate clearance and survival following injury. J Trauma 1993;35:584–8.

[57] McNelis J, Marini CP, Jurkiewicz A, et al. Prolonged lactate clearance is associated with increased mortality in the surgical intensive care unit. Am J Surg 2001;182:481–5.

[58] Nguyen HB, Rivers EP, Knoblich BP, et al. Early lactate clearance is associated with improved outcome in severe sepsis and septic shock. Crit Care Med 2004;32:1637–42.

[59] James JH, Luchette FA, McCarter FD, et al. Lactate is an unreliable indicator of tissue hypoxia in injury or sepsis. Lancet 1999;354:505–8.

[60] Luchette FA, Jenkins WA, Friend LA, et al. Hypoxia is not the sole cause of lactate production during shock. J Trauma 2002;52:415–9.

[61] Constant JS, Feng JJ, Zabel DD, et al. Lactate elicits vascular endothelial growth factor from macrophages: a possible alternative to hypoxia. Wound Repair Regen 2000;8: 353–60.

[62] James JH, Wagner KR, King JK, et al. Stimulation of both aerobic glycolysis and Na(+)-K(+)-ATPase activity in skeletal muscle by epinephrine or amylin. Am J Physiol 1999;277: E176–86.

[63] Clausen T. Na+-K+ pump regulation and skeletal muscle contractility. Physiol Rev 2003; 83:1269–324.

[64] Schurr A. Lactate, glucose and energy metabolism in the ischemic brain [review]. Int J Mol Med 2002;10:131–6.

[65] Payne RS, Tseng MT, Schurr A. The glucose paradox of cerebral ischemia: evidence for corticosterone involvement. Brain Res 2003;971:9–17.

[66] Danzl DF, Pozos RS, Auerbach PS, et al. Multicenter hypothermia survey. Ann Emerg Med 1987;16:1042–55.

[67] Rosomoff HL. Protective effects of hypothermia against pathological processes of the nervous system. Ann N Y Acad Sci 1959;80:475–86.

[68] Mild therapeutic hypothermia to improve the neurologic outcome after cardiac arrest. N Engl J Med 2002;346:549–56.

[69] Bernard SA, Gray TW, Buist MD, et al. Treatment of comatose survivors of out-of-hospital cardiac arrest with induced hypothermia. N Engl J Med 2002;346:557–63.

[70] Holzer M, Bernard SA, Hachimi-Idrissi S, et al. Hypothermia for neuroprotection after cardiac arrest: systematic review and individual patient data meta-analysis. Crit Care Med 2005;33:414–8.

[71] Marion DW, Leonov Y, Ginsberg M, et al. Resuscitative hypothermia. Crit Care Med 1996;24:S81–9.

[72] Nolan JP, Morley PT, Vanden Hoek TL, et al. Therapeutic hypothermia after cardiac arrest: an advisory statement by the advanced life support task force of the International Liaison Committee on Resuscitation. Circulation 2003;108:118–21.

[73] Merchant RM, Soar J, Skrifvars MB, et al. Therapeutic hypothermia utilization among physicians after resuscitation from cardiac arrest. Crit Care Med 2006;34(7): 1935–40.

[74] Tisherman SA. Hypothermia and injury. Curr Opin Crit Care 2004;10:512–9.

[75] Meyer DM, Horton JW. Effect of moderate hypothermia in the treatment of canine hemorrhagic shock. Ann Surg 1988;207:462–9.

[76] Crippen D, Safar P, Porter L, et al. Improved survival of hemorrhagic shock with oxygen and hypothermia in rats. Resuscitation 1991;21:271–81.

[77] Leonov Y, Safar P, Sterz F, et al. Extending the golden hour of hemorrhagic shock tolerance with oxygen plus hypothermia in awake rats. An exploratory study. Resuscitation 2002;52:193–202.

[78] Prueckner S, Safar P, Kentner R, et al. Mild hypothermia increases survival from severe pressure-controlled hemorrhagic shock in rats. J Trauma 2001;50:253–62.

[79] Wu X, Kochanek PM, Cochran K, et al. Mild hypothermia improves survival after prolonged, traumatic hemorrhagic shock in pigs. J Trauma 2005;59:291–9.

[80] Mizushima Y, Wang P, Cioffi WG, et al. Should normothermia be restored and maintained during resuscitation after trauma and hemorrhage? J Trauma 2000;48:58–65.

[81] Schreiber MA. Coagulopathy in the trauma patient. Curr Opin Crit Care 2005;11:590–7.

[82] Gubler KD, Gentilello LM, Hassantash SA, et al. The impact of hypothermia on dilutional coagulopathy. J.Trauma 1994;36:847–51.

[83] Rohrer MJ, Natale AM. Effect of hypothermia on the coagulation cascade. Crit Care Med 1992;20:1402–5.

[84] Watts DD, Trask A, Soeken K, et al. Hypothermic coagulopathy in trauma: effect of varying levels of hypothermia on enzyme speed, platelet function, and fibrinolytic activity. J Trauma 1998;44:846–54.

[85] Wolberg AS, Meng ZH, Monroe DM III, et al. A systematic evaluation of the effect of temperature on coagulation enzyme activity and platelet function. J Trauma 2004;56: 1221–8.

[86] Lee KR, Chung SP, Park IC, et al. Effect of induced and spontaneous hypothermia on survival time of uncontrolled hemorrhagic shock rat model. Yonsei Med J 2002;43: 511–7.

[87] Resnick DK, Marion DW, Darby JM. The effect of hypothermia on the incidence of delayed traumatic intracerebral hemorrhage. Neurosurgery 1994;34:252–5.

[88] Torossian A, Ruehlmann S, Middeke M, et al. Mild preseptic hypothermia is detrimental in rats. Crit Care Med 2004;32:1899–903.

[89] Hashiguchi N, Shiozaki T, Ogura H, et al. Mild hypothermia reduces expression of heat shock protein 60 in leukocytes from severely head-injured patients. J Trauma 2003;55: 1054–60.

[90] Rhee PM, Acosta J, Bridgeman A, et al. Survival after emergency department thoracotomy: review of published data from the past 25 years. J Am Coll Surg 2000;190:288–98.

[91] Bellamy R, Safar P, Tisherman SA, et al. Suspended animation for delayed resuscitation. Crit Care Med 1996;24:S24–47.

[92] Behringer W, Prueckner S, Safar P, et al. Rapid induction of mild cerebral hypothermia by cold aortic flush achieves normal recovery in a dog outcome model with 20-minute exsanguination cardiac arrest. Acad Emerg Med 2000;7:1341–8.

[93] Behringer W, Safar P, Wu X, et al. Survival without brain damage after clinical death of 60–120 mins in dogs using suspended animation by profound hypothermia. Crit Care Med 2003;31:1523–31.

[94] Wu X, Drabek T, Kochanek PM, et al. Induction of profound hypothermia for emergency preservation and resuscitation allows intact survival after cardiac arrest resulting from prolonged lethal hemorrhage and trauma in dogs. Circulation 2006;113:1974–82.

[95] Gregory JS, Flancbaum L, Townsend MC, et al. Incidence and timing of hypothermia in trauma patients undergoing operations. J Trauma 1991;31:795–8.

[96] Bernabei AF, Levison MA, Bender JS. The effects of hypothermia and injury severity on blood loss during trauma laparotomy. J Trauma 1992;33:835–9.

[97] Jurkovich GJ, Greiser WB, Luterman A, et al. Hypothermia in trauma victims: an ominous predictor of survival. J Trauma 1987;27:1019–24.

[98] Luna GK, Maier RV, Pavlin EG, et al. Incidence and effect of hypothermia in seriously injured patients. J Trauma 1987;27:1014–8.

[99] Martin RS, Kilgo PD, Miller PR, et al. Injury-associated hypothermia: an analysis of the 2004 National Trauma Data Bank. Shock 2005;24:114–8.

[100] Shafi S, Elliott AC, Gentilello L. Is hypothermia simply a marker of shock and injury severity or an independent risk factor for mortality in trauma patients? Analysis of a large national trauma registry. J Trauma 2005;59:1081–5.

[101] Wang HE, Callaway CW, Peitzman AB, et al. Admission hypothermia and outcome after major trauma. Crit Care Med 2005;33:1296–301.

[102] Gentilello LM, Jurkovich GJ, Stark MS, et al. Is hypothermia in the victim of major trauma protective or harmful? A randomized, prospective study. Ann Surg 1997;226:439–47.

[103] Clifton GL, Miller ER, Choi SC, et al. Lack of effect of induction of hypothermia after acute brain injury. N Engl J Med 2001;344:556–63.

[104] Shiozaki T, Hayakata T, Taneda M, et al. A multicenter prospective randomized controlled trial of the efficacy of mild hypothermia for severely head injured patients with low intracranial pressure. Mild Hypothermia Study Group in Japan. J Neurosurg 2001;94:50–4.

[105] Henderson WR, Dhingra VK, Chittock DR, et al. Hypothermia in the management of traumatic brain injury. A systematic review and meta-analysis. Intensive Care Med 2003;29: 1637–44.

[106] McIntyre LA, Fergusson DA, Hebert PC, et al. Prolonged therapeutic hypothermia after traumatic brain injury in adults: a systematic review. JAMA 2003;289:2992–9.

[107] Polderman KH, Tjong Tjin JR, Peerdeman SM, et al. Effects of therapeutic hypothermia on intracranial pressure and outcome in patients with severe head injury. Intensive Care Med 2002;28:1563–73.
[108] Jiang JY, Xu W, Li WP, et al. Effect of long-term mild hypothermia or short-term mild hypothermia on outcome of patients with severe traumatic brain injury. J Cereb Blood Flow Metab 2006;26:771–6.
[109] Zhi D, Zhang S, Lin X. Study on therapeutic mechanism and clinical effect of mild hypothermia in patients with severe head injury. Surg Neurol 2003;59:381–5.

ELSEVIER
SAUNDERS

Anesthesiology Clin
25 (2007) 65–74

ANESTHESIOLOGY
CLINICS

Training and Assessment of Trauma Management: The Role of Simulation-Based Medical Education

Haim Berkenstadt, MD[a,b,*],
David Erez, EMT-P, MSc[b], Yaron Munz, MD[b,c],
Daniel Simon, MD[d], Amitai Ziv, MD[b,e]

[a]*Department of Anesthesiology and Intensive Care, Sheba Medical Center, Tel Hashomer,
Tel Aviv University, Sackler School of Medicine, Tel Aviv, Israel*
[b]*The Israel Center for Medical Simulation, Sheba Medical Center, Tel Hashomer,
Tel Aviv University, Sackler School of Medicine, Tel Aviv, Israel*
[c]*Department of Surgery and Transplantation, Sheba Medical Center, Tel Hashomer,
Tel Aviv University, Sackler School of Medicine, Tel Aviv, Israel*
[d]*Trauma Unit, Sheba Medical Center, Tel Hashomer, Tel Aviv University,
Sackler School of Medicine, Tel Aviv, Israel*
[e]*Patient Safety and Medical Education, Sheba Medical Center, Tel Hashomer,
Tel Aviv University, Sackler School of Medicine, Tel Aviv, Israel*

Simulation-based medical education

Simulation-based medical education (SBME) is a rapidly growing field in the training of health professional and medical teams [1,2]. Important driving forces for the integration of SBME in formal curriculum and evaluation include, among others

Demands to minimize risks to patients by optimizing the use of simulation-based training that avoids exposing patients to unnecessary risk [3]

Demands by animals' rights movements to avoid the use of live animals for training health care providers [4]

Economic considerations that have reduced patient accessibility for traditional bedside medical teaching [5]

* Corresponding author. The Israel Center for Medical Simulation, Sheba Medical Center, 52621 Tel Hashomer, Tel Aviv, Israel.
E-mail address: berken@netvision.net.il (H. Berkenstadt).

0889-8537/07/$ - see front matter © 2007 Elsevier Inc. All rights reserved.
doi:10.1016/j.atc.2006.11.004
anesthesiology.theclinics.com

Medico-legal and risk management demands for accountability and high
   safety/quality standards [3]
The need for objective and reliable performance/competence evaluation,
   in addition to the traditional cognitive/knowledge-based assessments

Furthermore, following the aviation industry [6], the medical simulation
industry is now producing improved and more realistic high-fidelity training
devices, which are expanding and opening new horizons for medical training
and education.

SBME offers the opportunity for task training in various medical and
surgical procedures, and provides a "hands-on" empiric educational modality, enabling controlled proactive exposure of trainees to both regular and
complex, uncommon clinical scenarios. SBME training is trainee-oriented
and conducted in a safe and "mistake-forgiving" environment, where
trainees can learn from their errors and training can be adjusted to the
trainees' needs and deficiencies [1]. SBME further supplies a unique opportunity for team training, an important contributing factor to enhanced patient safety, and seldom addressed in traditional medical education.
Training is performed without the ethically disturbing duality of patient
care and medical training associated with traditional bedside teaching. Another important benefit of SBME is the reproducible, standardized, objective setting it provides for both formative assessment (debriefing) [7,8] and
summative assessment (testing) [9,10].

A major component of SBME, regardless of the simulation modality
used, is the ability to observe and record easily, and then debrief, the simulation session. During the debriefing session, participants get feedback from
peers and trainers on their clinical medical performance and nontechnical
skills. In most simulation centers, video recordings of training are used
for debriefing; this tool provides the participants the opportunity to see their
personal performance and how it affects the team performance, when relevant. From an educational point of view, the debriefing session may be
the most important part of the SBME experience, because it gives the par-
ticipant the possibility of reflecting on behavior and receiving feedback [11].

These potential benefits of SBME are relevant for the training and evaluation of trauma care in the prehospital and hospital environments, for
mass casualties, and in nonconventional warfare conditions. In this article,
the use of various simulation modalities, including simulated patients (role-
play actors), skills trainers, and computerized patient simulators in trauma
care training are reviewed.

Simulated patients

Objective Structured Clinical Examination using standardized simulated
patients is a widely used model of medical education [1,2]. Using this tool,
trainees are trained and evaluated on their ability to a take patient history,

perform a physical examination, communicate with the patient, and suggest appropriate treatment options. This simulation modality is used widely by medical and nursing schools and by medical boards worldwide, including the National Board of Medical Examiners in the United States, which recently introduced mandatory simulation-based clinical skills examinations as part of its requirements for a medical license in the United States [12]. These examinations reflect a major shift in the field of medical accreditation and licensure by acknowledging the crucial role of performance assessment in professional accreditation. This simulation modality was also adopted by the American College of Surgeons as one of the training and evaluation tools used in its Advanced Trauma Life Support (ATLS) course. This course was developed in an effort to standardize and improve trauma care, thereby increasing the consistency of medical treatment to trauma casualties [13]. Several studies have demonstrated the benefit of simulated patient–based evaluation of trauma management skills and the difference between this modality and cognitive knowledge assessment using a written standardized multiple choice examination [14,15].

Skills training

The use of task training simulators for the teaching of technical skills has become common in many fields of medicine, and demonstrates a reasonably good transfer of skills from models to humans [16–19]. In the training of trauma care, various skills trainers are used for teaching novices trauma-related procedures like chest drain insertion, cricothyroidotomy, and focused abdominal sonography for trauma (FAST). The emergency insertion of a chest drain for tension pneumothorax or hemothorax following trauma is considered to be safe when performed by trained physicians [20]. However, the use of live animals to train novices to perform this procedure is prohibited because of increasing pressure from animals' rights movements in a growing number of countries, such as the United Kingdom. Therefore, alternatives such as models of thoracic drainage based on animal cadaveric models have been developed [21]. Recently, the American College of Surgeons accepted the TraumaMan simulator (Simulab Corporation, Seattle, Washington) [22] as an alternative to the ATLS animal surgical skill station. In a recent validation study, following chest drain insertion to the Trauma-Man simulator, experienced ATLS instructors recommended the simulator to train novice physicians in this procedure [23]. In the same study, 42 novice participants of the ATLS course trained with both animal skills laboratory and the simulator found the simulator superior to the animal model in teaching anatomic landmarks. This finding is crucial for teaching the procedural steps, especially in view of a recent survey demonstrating that 45% of the junior physicians surveyed would have placed the chest drain outside the safe insertion triangle [24].

In another critical life-saving procedure, similar findings were reported for cricothyroidotomy [25,26]. Simulation modalities were used to assess the success rate by novices in performing the procedure, and its learning curve. In one simulation-based evaluation, a 100% success rate in achieving an adequate airway within acceptable time limits was found [27], and training for five attempts at least, or until cricothyroidotomy time was 40 seconds or less, was recommended [28]. Unfortunately, neither study assessed the transference of skills from the simulation modalities to humans, and conclusions are limited to the skills trainer.

Lately, a training program for the performance of FAST by nonradiologists (surgeons, emergency physicians, and trauma anesthesiologists) using the UltraSim simulator (MedSim, Israel) [29] was developed and validated [30]. The FAST examination allows for rapid bedside diagnosis of intra-abdominal, pleural, or pericardial hemorrhage in trauma casualties, even in the prehospital setting when radiologists are not available [31]. The simulation-based curriculum improved the correct transducer placement and the quality of the images obtained, shortened the time required for obtaining images, and increased the incidence of correct diagnosis. Construct validity, namely the ability of the simulation training program and the assessment tools to differentiate among participants according to their experience in performing the task, was demonstrated and participants recommended using this training modality for all trauma physicians.

Computerized patient simulators

Computerized patient simulators, based on a mannequin connected to a physiologic monitor and run by a computerized system located in the relevant clinical environment, can be programmed for diverse clinical scenarios and can permit a safe and reproducible training environment. This type of simulation-based training requires physicians to identify problems and provide solutions, as if it were a real emergency situation (ie, infuse fluids, perform orotracheal intubation, or insert a thorax drain). For example, while using the Human Patient Simulator or the Emergency Care Simulator (Medical Education Technologies, METI, Sarasota, Florida) [32], the treating physician can talk to the mannequin and get an answer from the operator through a speaker in the mannequin's head; check pupils (which react to light); feel arterial pulses; listen to cardiac and lung sounds; and collect information on heart rate, blood pressure, respiratory rate, and oxygen saturation. Medications and fluids can be administered to the simulator, which responds appropriately, based on an interaction between the mannequin's current underlying physiology and the dose and the pharmacokinetics and pharmacodynamics of the medication. In addition, a number of procedures like airway management, cricothyroidotomy, and chest drain insertion can be performed on the mannequin. The SimMan simulator (Laerdal, Norway)

[33] is similar with respect to airway, breathing, and circulation management, but the pupils are not interactive and the mannequin does not have preprogrammed physiologic responses to medications or treatments, although these responses can be simulated through the mannequin's computer interface. The AirMan simulator (Laerdal, Norway) is designed to provide a platform for training airway management.

Advanced medical simulation has been used in a number of medical fields to improve training, clinical performance, and competence assessment, and in emergency room or operating room resource management training [1,34]. Advanced simulation has also been used for learning about errors made during critical emergency situations, and understanding the patterns of human errors during anesthesia, thus providing recommendations for changes in teaching and education [35,36]. In trauma care, advanced simulation has been incorporated into the training programs of medics, paramedics, physicians, and medical teams worldwide, mainly by military training programs. For example, advanced simulation has been introduced for the training of basic trauma-related skills for military emergency personnel [37], and to evaluate the competence of surgery interns after a standard ATLS course [38]. Although the face validity of such training is high, and there are high expectations for this training modality [39], validation of simulation-based training in trauma management is limited. The construct validity of advanced simulation in the training of emergency medicine scenarios was demonstrated by Gordon and colleagues [40], and the value of advanced simulation in promoting trauma management was demonstrated [41,42].

Medical simulation was used also to identify deficiencies in the stabilization of children presenting to emergency departments, revealing that mistakes, including estimating a child's weight, preparing for intraosseous needle placement, ordering intravenous fluid boluses, and applying warming measures, are ubiquitous [43]. In another study, the findings of major deviations in airway management, and in the evaluation of secondary respiratory and hemodynamic deterioration in the intubated trauma patient, were followed by changes in the training curriculum and, as a consequence, improvement in performance [44]. These findings of performance improvement after changes in curriculum are not trivial in view of the limited data published supporting the beneficial effects of simulation-based training. The report by Chopra and colleagues [45] demonstrated the positive effect of simulation training on the subsequent management of similar critical incidents, but Olympio and colleagues [46] failed to demonstrate the influence of simulation training on the management of esophageal intubation. However, the suggested beneficial effect of simulation-based airway management training is supported by a recent prospective, randomized, controlled study, which demonstrated that simulator training independently improved scores achieved by interns treating trauma-related scenarios after graduating from a 1-day trauma course, compared with training based on moulage patients [47].

Team training

One of the major applications of SBME in the training of trauma management is its use in team training. Although surgical, anesthesiology, and emergency medicine trainees receive feedback on their technical performance from their trainers, they rarely receive feedback on their nontechnical or team skills. The importance of nontechnical skills is highlighted by data from aviation, demonstrating that 70% of errors have human causes and that a large number of errors are a result of failures in interpersonal communication, decision making, and leadership [48]. Further support comes from the finding that errors in the operating theater are rarely caused by deficiencies in technical performance [49]. They result more from impaired decision making, an absence of situation awareness, and failures in interpersonal communication.

These similarities between surgery, anesthesiology, and trauma management, and aviation characteristics, led to the adoption of the concept of crew resource management from aviation, and courses in crisis management for anesthesiologists and surgical teams based on the crew resource management concept were developed [50–52]. These crew resource management courses were demonstrated to reduce the risks of serious and life-threatening events in medicine and aviation [53,54]. These courses involve various tools and methods for team training, including lectures; video-based discussion of the aspects of poor and good communication, teamwork, and leadership; skill stations on teamwork skills (for example, inline stabilization for endotracheal intubation); and interactive discussions on trauma case management and triage. However, a full-scale simulation scenario followed by a video-based debriefing seems to be the ultimate training tool.

One of the reasons for the apparent failure to make nontechnical skills a focus of training among medical specialties has been the difficulty encountered in the objective assessment of these skills to enable structured feedback. Even in Israel, where a joint effort by the Israeli Defense Forces Medical Corps and the Israel Center for Medical Simulation promoted simulation-based training of prehospital military medical teams to the level of standard in recent years, training is focused mainly on technical performance. Efforts in the direction of nontechnical skills assessment are being made by the authors and by other groups in the fields of surgery [55] and anesthesiology [56].

Web-based teaching

In any modality of SBME, it is useful to provide participants with associated theoretic material in advance of their simulation-based training, to achieve a more homogeneous group by triggering prior knowledge, and stressing important learning points [11]. One of the options is to use web-based teaching tools, such as the "HighLearn" [57], to facilitate learning the cognitive knowledge relevant for training, while incorporating tasks and examinations for the trainees.

Practical aspects

SBME is used increasingly for training medical personnel in trauma care. It is important to recognize the broad spectrum of simulation modalities and devices and to use simulation in a cost-effective manner, while recognizing the SBME's limitations and adjusting the training program and the simulation tools to the target population and the educational goals. Simulation technologies should supplement, not replace, the traditional methods of teaching cognitive knowledge. For example

The cognitive aspects of the teaching module can be taught by the traditional methods of lectures and self-guided learning before partaking in the simulation training.

The acquisition and practice of technical skills, such as chest drain insertion and airway management skills, can be performed on task trainer simulators like the TraumaMan and the AirMan.

Teamwork skills like inline stabilization of the spine can be trained before the team participates in a full trauma drill.

Computerized simulators can be used for full-scale, high-fidelity simulation scenarios, and video recordings of the training can be used for debriefing team work and other aspects of performance.

Summary

Simulation-based medical simulation offers a safe and "mistake-forgiving" environment to teach and train medical professionals. The diverse range of medical simulation modalities enables trainees to acquire and practice an array of tasks and skills. SBME offers the field of trauma training multiple opportunities to enhance the effectiveness of the education provided in this challenging domain. Further research is needed to better learn the role of simulation-based learning in trauma management and education.

References

[1] Issenberg SB, McGaghie WC, Hart IR, et al. Simulation technology for health care professional skills training and assessment. JAMA 1999;282(9):861–6.

[2] Ziv A, Small S, Wolpe P. Patient safety and simulation based medical education. Med Teach 2000;22(5):489–95.

[3] Committee on Quality of Health Care in America, Institute of Medicine To err is human: building a safer health system. Kohn LT, Corrigan JM, Donaldson MS, editors. Washington, DC: Institute of Medicine, National Academy Press; 2000. p. 312.

[4] Cohen C. The case for the use of animals in biomedical research. N Engl J Med 1986;315: 865–70.

[5] The Israel National Institute for Health Policy and Health Services Research. Curriculum for medical schools towards the 21st century. Jerusalem (Israel): The Israel National Institute for Health Policy and Health Services Research; 2002.

[6] Helmreich RL, Davies JM. Anaesthetic simulation and lessons to be learned from aviation. Can J Anaesth 1997;44(9):907–12.

[7] Ende J. Feedback in clinical medical education. JAMA 1983;250(6):777–81.

[8] Rooks L, Watson RT, Harris JO. A primary care preceptorship for first-year medical students coordinated by an area health education center program: a six-year review. Acad Med 2001;76(5):489–92.

[9] MacRae H, Regehr G, Leadbetter W, et al. A comprehensive examination for senior surgical residents. Am J Surg 2000;179(3):190–3.

[10] Weller JM, Bloch M, Young S, et al. Evaluation of high fidelity patient simulator in assessment of performance of anaesthetists. Br J Anaesth 2003;90(1):43–7.

[11] Østergaard HT, Østergaard D, Lippert A. Implementation of team training in medical education in Denmark. Qual Saf Health Care 2004;13(Suppl):i91–5.

[12] Papadakis MA. The step 2 clinical skills examination. N Engl J Med 2004;350(17): 1703–5.

[13] van Olden GD, Meeuwis JD, Bolhuis HW, et al. Clinical impact of advanced trauma life support. Am J Emerg Med 2004;22(7):522–5.

[14] Ali J, Adam R, Pierre I, et al. Comparison of performance two years after the old and new (interactive) ATLS courses. J Surg Res 2001;97(1):71–5.

[15] Ali J, Adam RU, Josa D, et al. Comparison of performance of interns completing the old (1993) and new interactive (1997) Advanced Trauma Life Support courses. J Trauma 1999;46(1):80–6.

[16] Anastakis DJ, Regehr G, Reznick RK, et al. Assessment of technical skills transfer from the bench training model to the human model. Am J Surg 1999;177(2):167–70.

[17] Ost D, DeRosiers A, Britt EJ, et al. Assessment of a bronchoscopy simulator. Am J Respir Crit Care Med 2001;164(12):2248–55.

[18] Grantcharov TP, Kristiansen VB, Bendix J, et al. Randomized clinical trial of virtual reality simulation for laparoscopic skills training. Br J Surg 2004;91(2):146–50.

[19] Adrales GL, Park AE, Chu UB, et al. A valid method of laparoscopic simulation training and competence assessment. J Surg Res 2003;114(2):156–62.

[20] Collop NA, Kim S, Sahn SA. Analysis of tube thoracostomy performed by pulmonologists at a teaching hospital. Chest 1997;112(3):709–13.

[21] Eaton BD, Messent DO, Haywood IR. Animal cadaveric models for advanced trauma life support training. Ann R Coll Surg Engl 1990;72(2):135–9.

[22] Simulab Corporation. Available at: http://www.simulab.com/.

[23] Berkenstadt H, Munz Y, Trodler G, et al. Evaluation of the trauma-man® simulator for training in chest drain insertion. Eur J Trauma 2006;32:523–6.

[24] Griffiths JR, Roberts N. Do junior doctors know where to insert chest drains safely? Postgrad Med J 2005;81(957):456–8.

[25] Isaacs JH Jr, Pedersen AD. Emergency cricothyroidotomy. Am Surg 1997;63(4):346–9.

[26] Leibovici D, Fredman B, Gofrit ON, et al. Prehospital cricothyroidotomy by physicians. Am J Emerg Med 1997;15(1):91–3.

[27] Vadodaria BS, Gandhi SD, McIndoe AK. Comparison of four different emergency airway access equipment sets on a human patient simulator. Anaesthesia 2004;59(1): 73–9.

[28] Wong DT, Prabhu AJ, Coloma M, et al. What is the minimum training required for successful cricothyroidotomy?: a study in mannequins. Anesthesiology 2003;98(2):349–53.

[29] MedSim Advanced Medical Simulation. Available at: http://www.medsim.com/.

[30] Kapelian I, Simon D, Ziv A, et al. The use of simulation for focused abdominal sonography in trauma (FAST) training. Presented at the 17th Annual Meeting of the Israeli Trauma Society. Herzelia, Israel, September 2005.

[31] Walcher F, Weinlich M, Conrad G, et al. Prehospital ultrasound imaging improves management of abdominal trauma. Br J Surg 2006;93(2):238–42.

[32] Medical Education Technologies, Inc. Available at: http://www.meti.com/.

[33] Laerdal. Available at: http://www.laerdal.com/.

[34] Gaba DM. Improving anesthesiologists' performance by simulating reality. Anesthesiology 1992;76(4):491–4.

[35] Schwid HA, O'Donnell D. Anesthesiologists' management of simulated critical incidents. Anesthesiology 1992;76(4):495–501.

[36] De-Anda A, Gaba DM. Unplanned incidents during comprehensive anesthesia simulation. Anesth Analg 1990;71:77–82.

[37] Treloar D, Hawayek J, Montgomery JR, et al. On site and distance education of emergency personnel with a human patient simulator. Mil Med 2001;166(1):103–6.

[38] Ali J, Gana TJ, Howard M. Trauma mannequin assessment of management skills of surgical residents after advanced trauma life support training. J Surg Res 2000;93(1):197–200.

[39] Barsuk D, Berkenstadt H, Stein M, et al. [Advanced patient simulators in pre-hospital trauma management training–the trainees' perspective]. Harefuah 2003;142(2):87–90 [in Hebrew].

[40] Gordon JA, Tancredi D, Binder W, et al. Assessing global performance in emergency medicine using high fidelity patient simulator: a pilot study. Acad Emerg Med 2003;78(10 Suppl): S45–7.

[41] Marshall RL, Smith JS, Gorman P, et al. Use of a human patient simulator in the development of resident trauma management skills. J Trauma 2001;51(1):17–21.

[42] Lee SK, Pardo M, Gaba D, et al. Trauma assessment training with a patient simulator: a prospective, randomized study. J Trauma 2003;55(4):651–7.

[43] Hunt EA, Hohenhaus SM, Luo X, et al. Simulation of pediatric trauma stabilization in 35 North Carolina emergency departments: identification of targets for performance improvement. Pediatrics 2006;117(3):641–8.

[44] Barsuk D, Ziv A, Lin G, et al. Using advanced simulation for recognition and correction of gaps in airway and breathing management skills in prehospital trauma care. Anesth Analg 2005;100(3):803–9.

[45] Chopra V, Gesink BJ, de Jong J, et al. Does training on an anaesthesia simulator lead to improvement in performance? Br J Anaesth 1994;73(3):293–7.

[46] Olympio MA, Whelan R, Ford RP, et al. Failure of simulation training to change residents' management of oesophageal intubation. Br J Anaesth 2003;91(3):312–8.

[47] Block EF, Lottenberg I, Flint L, et al. Use of human patient simulator for the advanced trauma life support course. Am Surg 2002;68(7):648–51.

[48] Helmreich RL, Merritt AC, Wilhelm JA. The evolution of crew resource management training in commercial aviation. Int J Aviat Psychol 1999;9:19–32.

[49] Chopra V, Bovill JG, Spierdijk J, et al. Reported significant observations during anaesthesia: a prospective analysis over an 18-month period. Br J Anaesth 1992;68:13–7.

[50] Howard SK, Gaba DM, Fish KJ, et al. Anesthesia crisis resource management training: teaching anesthesiologists to handle critical incidents. Aviat Space Environ Med 1992; 63(9):763–70.

[51] Holzman RS, Cooper JB, Gaba DM, et al. Anesthesia crisis resource management: real-life simulation training in operating room crises. J Clin Anesth 1995;7:675–87.

[52] Shapiro MJ, Morey JC, Small SD, et al. Simulation based teamwork training for emergency department staff: does it improve clinical team performance when added to an existing didactic teamwork curriculum? Qual Saf Health Care 2004;13(6):417–21.

[53] Morey J, Simon R, Jay G, et al. Error reduction and performance improvement in the emergency department through formal teamwork training: evaluation results of the MedTeams project. Health Serv Res 2002;37(6):1553–81.

[54] O'Connor P, Flin R, Fletcher G. Techniques used to evaluate crew resource management training: a literature review. Human Factors in Aerospace Safety 2002;2:217–33.

[55] Moorthy K, Munz Y, Adams S, et al. A human factors analysis of technical and team skills among surgical trainees during procedural simulations in a simulated operating theatre. Ann Surg 2005;242(5):631–9.
[56] Fletcher G, Flin R, McGeorge P, et al. Anaesthetists' Non-Technical Skills (ANTS): evaluation of a behavioural marker system. Br J Anaesth 2003;90:580–8.
[57] Britannica Knowledge Systems. Available at: http://www.britannica-ks.com/.

ELSEVIER
SAUNDERS

Anesthesiology Clin
25 (2007) 75–90

ANESTHESIOLOGY
CLINICS

Geriatric Trauma: Special Considerations in the Anesthetic Management of the Injured Elderly Patient

Michael C. Lewis, MD[a],*, Karim Abouelenin, MD[a], Miguel Paniagua, MD[b]

[a]Department of Anesthesiology, Miller School of Medicine at the
University of Miami, Miami, FL 33101, USA
[b]Miami GRECC, VA Medical Center, Department of Geriatrics,
Miller School of Medicine at the University of Miami, Miami, FL 33125, USA

Traumatic injury is the foremost cause of mortality in patients aged over 44 years [1]. At the end of the twentieth century, almost 20% of injuries occurred in the elderly population [2]. These patients are susceptible to a distinctive injury pattern. They respond differently to trauma, recover more slowly [3], and have higher morbidity and mortality [4]. It is not clear if these differences are due to increased comorbidity [4] or decreased physiologic reserve.

After traumatic injury, it is important that all interventions be evidence based. There are few prospective randomized controlled trials that focus on elderly issues, and within the published studies there is no uniform definition of the term "elderly." Therefore, many of the recommendations may not be applicable. Despite these limitations, this article aims to draw conclusions from the available literature. Where possible, it makes recommendations as to the optimal anesthetic management of elderly trauma patients.

Aging

Senescence results in a progressive decline in cellular function, resulting in a loss of organ performance. Cells lose their capacity to respond to injury

* Corresponding author. Department of Anesthesiology, Jackson Memorial Hospital, 1611 NW 12th Ave., Miami, FL 33136.
  E-mail address: mclewis@med.miami.edu (M.C. Lewis).

0889-8537/07/$ - see front matter © 2007 Elsevier Inc. All rights reserved.
doi:10.1016/j.atc.2006.11.002   *anesthesiology.theclinics.com*

and eventually die. Aging, therefore, is a progressive process depicted as maintenance of life with a diminishing capability for adjustment [5]. It is associated with impaired adaptive and homeostatic mechanisms, resulting in an increased susceptibility to the effects of stress. Function may seem to be unchanged, yet physiologic reserve diminishes. Any disruption of homeostasis that is well tolerated by younger adults might precipitate functional decline in the elderly population. The situation is further compounded by variable response to medications and comorbidity.

Definition: the geriatric trauma patient

Historically, the term "elderly" was applied to individuals over 65 years of age. However, aging is now viewed as a physiologic continuum rather than chronologic age.

It may be more useful to divide the geriatric population into "young old," which includes individuals between the ages of 65 and 80 years, and "Oldest-old," which includes individuals over 80 years of age. Geriatric trauma patients fare worse than their younger counterparts [6,7]. The prognosis in the octogenarian group is significantly worse.

Physiologic changes in the elderly population

Cardiac function declines by 50% between the ages of 20 and 80 years. This impaired cardiac function, paired with decreased sensitivity to catecholamines (and possibly overlaid with β-blocker therapy), complicates the management of the hemodynamically compromised older patient.

Above the age of 50 years, renal mass is lost, with a corresponding fall in glomerular filtration rate [8,9].

Respiratory function is compromised in the elderly population. There is an observed loss of the lung elastic recoil and significant reduction of the vital capacity. These changes result in dependence on diaphragmatic breathing, impaired mucociliary clearance of bacteria, and reduced ability to cough [10]. There is a disruption of the normal matching of ventilation and perfusion. Forced expiratory volume in 1 second, forced vital capacity, and peak expiratory flow rate are decreased [11]. Such changes in diffusion capacity alterations in ventilation–perfusion mismatch [12] and in closing volumes mean that there is a decrease in baseline arterial oxygen tension with age [13]. Alterations in compliance result in an increased work of breathing [14]. The combination of these factors means that there is an increased risk of respiratory failure in the elderly patient, resulting in a higher incidence of mechanical ventilation, [15] acute lung injury, and ventilation-associated pneumonia as a consequence of longer ICU stay and high morbidity.

There are age-related changes of endocrine function. The tissue responsiveness to thyroxin and its production is reduced with aging [16]. Secretion of cortisol does not seem to change with aging [17].

Functional reserve

When an organism maintains a steady state in the face of increased physiologic demand, it is said to demonstrate a good functional reserve. Fig. 1 illustrates this divergence between "baseline" and "stress" situations. Imbalance within the system therefore results in a breakdown of homeostatic compensation. A decline in functional reserve may in the elderly patient precipitate a serious decline in performance when the elderly patient is exposed to stress and increases the risk of age-related disease.

Because of decreasing functional reserve, the older patient is less able to preserve homeostasis in face of such a physical insult [18]. There is inconsistency in this decline in functional reserve. The variability is rooted within lifestyle choices, environmental factors, genetics, and the presence of age-related disease. Older trauma victims do not cope as well as younger adults [19,20]. Often, aggressive treatment is less likely to be received by the older patient [21]. Consequently, elderly trauma victims are less able to preserve sufficient perfusion of vital organs [22]. After injury, elderly patients are more likely to arrive in the emergency department in hypotensive shock and to be hypothermic. This decreased functional reserve contributes to the higher percentage of the geriatric trauma victims that appear in the early trauma mortality statistics. It affects infection-related deaths and multiple organ dysfunction syndromes.

Diminished reserve, manifested as comorbid disease states, seems to have a negative predictive value for outcome [23]. However, when aggressive treatment is initiated, the outcome difference between younger and older adult diminishes [24]. When there is an aggressive approach to management, age does not necessarily contribute to negative outcome [25].

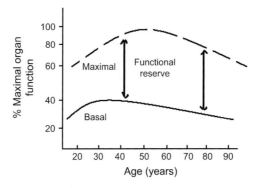

Fig. 1. The functional reserve is the difference between basal function (*solid line*) and maximal function (*broken line*). Even in healthy individuals, this functional reserve is reduced. (*From* Muravchick S. Geroanesthesia: principles for management of the elderly patient. St. Louis (MO): Mosby 1997; with permission.)

Mechanisms of injury

There is a higher risk of chest injuries in the elderly population [26]. Older drivers have a higher incidence of rib and sternal fractures [27]. Rib fractures or flail chest may sometimes occur in elderly persons without the significant underlying pulmonary contusion that would be anticipated in a younger patient [28]. There seem to be increases in fractures of the vertebrae, the hip, and the distal forearm, attributed to a high prevalence of osteoporosis [29].

In contrast to the younger adult trauma patient, the elderly victim is less likely to die as a direct result of their accident. Death is often associated with comorbidity, functional decline, and postoperative complications [30].

Dramatic accidents are not the most common reason why elderly patients present to the trauma unit. The commonest mechanism of injury is the fall [31,32]. Various factors predispose elderly persons to falls, such as unsteady gait, orthostatic hypotension, and slow reaction time [33]. Falls can lead to significant injuries [34]. It has been estimated that falls can account for over 50% of traumatic deaths [35]. Patients who have severe injuries despite a seemingly minor mechanism of injury are more likely to be older than 55 years of age [36], and the death rate is especially high in octogenarians [37].

Traffic accidents involving drivers or pedestrians are the second and third most common cause of injuries in the elderly population, respectively [31]. Underlying disease, decreases in hearing or vision, muscle weakness, and reduced reaction times [38] are contributing factors [39].

Thermal injuries occur more frequently in the elderly population. This increased risk could be attributable to a reduced sense of smell, impaired hearing or vision, or reduced mobility and reaction time. These injuries are inclined to be more serious in terms of surface area and depth [40]. The propensity to more severe thermal injury may be attributable to age-related alterations in skin morphology and diminished visual, olfactory, and auditory senses.

Elder mistreatment should be considered when evaluating the injured older patient. Investigations suggest that in excess of 2% of elders are abused or neglected [41,42].

Initial pre-hospital evaluation: triage and treatment

Limited physiologic reserve means that the prognosis of the elderly injured patient is much better when the patient is rapidly transported to a trauma center [43,44]. Despite this observation, there is a significant absence of rapid triage of elderly patients to established trauma centers

Which patients should receive aggressive therapy?

It is important to recognize early patients in whom aggressive additional resuscitation is futile. Measures of physiologic derangement may be used to identify such patients and differentiate them from those who might benefit from aggressive resuscitation strategies. It has been suggested that particular awareness is needed when triaging elderly trauma victims because their injuries may be hidden, thus putting them at risk for admission to a level of care that may be unsuitable given the degree of their injuries [45].

There is evidence of the predictive value on mortality of the Revised Trauma Score (Table 1). A specific numerical score predicting mortality has not been found [46]. One observer noted 100% mortality when the initial respiratory rate was less than 10 breaths per minute [47].

The adequacy of resuscitation may be estimated using the arterial base deficit. In the elderly patient, even a minor base deficit may have significant negative predictive value [48]. Base deficit may help identify a subgroup of patients that would possibly benefit from intensive resuscitative efforts.

The Injury Severity Score (ISS) is an anatomic scoring system (Table 2) that gives a global score for patients who have multiple injuries. It has been shown to be a strong predictor of mortality in geriatric patients [49]. The ISS has limited prognostic capabilities in geriatric trauma because of significant delays in obtaining the data to calculate the scores.

One modification of the ISS is the Geriatric Trauma Survival Score [50]. The Geriatric Trauma Survival Score uses the ISS, patient age, and the absence of cardiac symptoms or septic complications to predict outcome. It has not been widely shown to predict survival [51].

Injury assessment and resuscitation

The primary survey in the geriatric patient is no different from that in the younger adult.

Airway

The airway can be physically obstructed as a result of direct injury, edema, or foreign bodies. Patients may not be able to protect the airway if there is a decreased level of consciousness. Either case might necessitate endotracheal

Table 1
Determination of the Revised Trauma Score

Glasgow Coma Scale	Systolic blood pressure (mm Hg)	Respiratory rate	Coded value
13–15	>89	10–29	4
9–12	76–89	>29	3
6–8	50–75	6–9	2
4–5	1–49	1–5	1
3	0	0	0

The Revised Trauma Score is a physiologic scoring system. It is scored from the first set of data obtained. *Adapted from* Champion HR, Sacco WJ, Copes WS. A revision of the trauma score. J Trauma 1989;29(5):623–9.

Table 2
Determination of the Injury Severity Score

Region	Injury description	Abbreviated injury scale	Square of top three	Injury Severity Score
Head and neck	Cerebral bleed	4	16	—
Face	Facial lacerations	1	—	—
Chest	Flail chest	4	16	—
Abdomen	Ruptured spleen	5	25	—
Extremity	Fractured radius	2	—	—
External	No injury	0	0	57

The three most severely injured body regions have their score squared and added together to produce the Injury Severity Score. *Adapted from* Baker SP, O'Neill B, Haddon W, et al. The injury severity score: a method for describing patients with multiple injuries and evaluating emergency care. J Trauma 1974;14:187–96.

intubation. Orotracheal intubation under anesthesia with planned neuromuscular blockade and in-line cervical alignment remains the safest and most effective method for airway control in the severely injured patient [52].

Recommendations concerning the doses of anesthesia medications used to facilitate intubation are shown in Table 3. In the older adult, the doses of many of the sedative agents used to facilitate intubation may have to be further altered. Their pharmacokinetics could be altered due to the trauma [53] or to physiologic changes associated with aging [13,54,55].

To avoid hypotension in the elderly trauma patient, the doses of the etomidate [56], barbiturates [57], and benzodiazepines [58,59] need to be reduced. For example, an 80-year-old trauma patient needs less than half the amount of etomidate to reach the same EEG endpoint as a 22-year-old patient [56]. This reduction of blood pressure in the elderly patient is especially marked when the patient is hypovolemic. Ketamine is commonly used in the trauma scenario. In the geriatric patient, this drug has a reduced clearance and is expected to have a longer duration of action.

The opioids have an increased activity or alterations in pharmacokinetics in the elderly patient. A reduction in the dosage of morphine [60], alfentanil, fentanyl [61], and remifentanil [62] is recommended. The only exception to

Table 3
Dosage alteration for the anesthetic drugs used to facilitate intubation in the elderly patient

Class of medication	Change of dose in the elderly patient
Sedatives	Reduction of 50% of bolus dose
Depolarizing neuromuscular blocking agent (succinylcholine)	No reduction in bolus dose
Nondepolarizing neuromuscular blocking agents	No reduction in bolus dose
Opioids	Reduction of 50% of bolus dose

this rule is meperidine, for which no changes in clearance rate or terminal elimination half-time value have been shown [63]. However, due to its CNS-active toxic metabolite, normeperidine, its use is not advocated in elderly patients.

In the geriatric population, a reduction in physical activity theoretically should result in a reduction in sensitivity due to up-regulation to neuromuscular blockers. In contrast, augmented exercise increases sensitivity to neuromuscular-blocking drugs receptors [50]. Clinically, the doses of neuromuscular blockers are usually unchanged [64].

There are a number of considerations for the initial airway management of the geriatric patient [65]. Because of a widespread loss of all muscular and neural elements, laryngeal structures undergo a gradual deterioration in function. Older patients exhibit a decrease in protective airway reflexes [66]. Aspiration is more common, and planning is required for its prevention. The elderly patient may be edentulous. Alternatively, there may be poor dentition, making damage to the teeth more likely [67]. Loose-fitting dentures should be removed. Visualization of the glottis is more difficult if there is poor mouth opening and stiffening of the atlanto-occipital joint [68]. If a neck immobilizer has been placed, then visualization of the cords may be difficult.

Breathing

Assessment of ventilation, as with all trauma patients, is accomplished by the look, listen, and feel approach. Confirmation is obtained by capnography and oximetry. The presence of a semi-rigid neck collar with suspected cervical neck injuries does not affect ventilation [69].

Chest injuries, such as rib fractures and pulmonary contusion, are common. Pulmonary contusion is considered to be one of the most common blunt thoracic injuries. Noninvasive ventilation via a continuous positive airway pressure mask has been described in the literature for the management of hypoxemia caused by lung contusion and for other medical conditions [34]. This effect may serve as a pathophysiologic-directed therapy for hypoxemic patients who have blunt chest injury in whom endotracheal intubation is not required.

Circulation

Significant reductions in coronary blood flow can occur in the absence of known coronary artery disease [69]. The aging myocardium is also less able to respond to circulating catecholamines [52]. Therefore, the hypovolemic geriatric patient may not develop tachycardia in the presence of hypovolemia. Elderly patients may also be taking medications such as β-blockers that alter their heart rate response. Often, geriatric patients have hypertension; therefore, a normal or borderline blood pressure should be treated with suspicion.

The elderly trauma victim as compared with their younger counterpart may be less able to compensate for changing oxygen demands by increasing cardiac output. They may be dependent on a level of circulating hemoglobin that should be kept at adequate levels [19].

Geriatric patients do not handle hypovolemia well, nor do they tolerate fluid overload. The consensus opinion is that initial fluid administration should be with crystalloid. Initially, a fluid challenge of 1 or 2 L should be given gradually and with caution [70]. If there is no significant improvement in vital signs, then blood should be administered. Because of the geriatric patient's decreased cardiac reserve, invasive monitoring should be considered once the decision to transfuse blood is made.

Sclalea and colleagues [103] initiated a practice recommendation of placing a pulmonary artery catheter in selected geriatric trauma patients (ie, patients who had systolic blood pressure of <130 mm Hg, acidosis, multiple fractures, head injury, and motor–pedestrian mechanism of injury). Scalea also recommended a limited evaluation phase in the trauma unit, after which the patient should be transferred to the ICU. When this principle was used with a mean time to optimization of 2.2 hours, survival was improved from 7% to 53%. Although this study has not been repeated, it draws our attention to the importance of early invasive monitoring in the elderly trauma patient.

Monitoring

A low threshold for early invasive monitoring initiation is used in elderly patients. This is important for the optimization of O_2 delivery.

Elderly trauma patients with physiologic compromise, significant injury, high-risk mechanism of injury, uncertain cardiovascular status, or chronic cardiovascular or renal disease should undergo invasive hemodynamic monitoring using a pulmonary artery catheter. Such early invasive monitoring has been associated with improved survival in the geriatric trauma patient [69]. It has been argued that patients who have a normal echocardiogram and EKG do not need invasive monitoring [71]. Evidence suggests that when such routine echocardiograms are introduced, they do little to change management; rather, they delay surgery [72]. Noninvasive hemodynamic monitoring in critically ill patients using bioimpedance technology has been shown to be a reliable alternative to invasive thermodilution techniques in geriatric trauma patients [73]. Recent studies have demonstrated that invasive intraoperative hemodynamic monitoring with fluid challenges during repair of femoral fracture under general anesthesia shortens the time to being medically fit for discharge [74].

A possible algorithm for the hemodynamic invasive monitoring of such elderly trauma patients has been developed (Fig. 2) [70]. If trauma is mild, there are no signs of hypoperfusion, and there is no significant systemic disease. Standard American Society of Anesthesiologists (ASA)

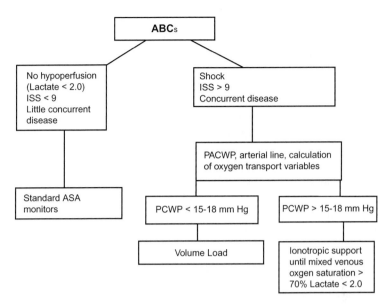

Fig. 2. An algorithm for the initial resuscitation of the elderly trauma victim. ISS, Injury Severity Score; PACWP, pulmonary artery capillary wedge pressure; PCWP, pulmonary capillary wedge pressure. The American Society of Anesthesiologists (ASA) has published minimal monitoring standards for patients undergoing general anesthesia. These standards call for monitoring of the patient's oxygenation (inspired gas and arterial saturation), ventilation (capnography), circulation (ECG, arterial blood pressure), and temperature (thermometer). (*Modified from* Santora TA, Schinco MA, Trooskin SZ. Management of TRAUMA in the elderly patient. Surg Clin North Am 1994;74;163–85; with permission.)

monitors would suffice. If the injury is greater than mild (ISS >9), if there are signs of shock or hypovolemia, and if the patient has significant systemic disease, an arterial line and pulmonary artery catheter (oximetry type preferably) should be inserted. Otherwise, oxygen transport variables need to be calculated. If the wedge pressure is low (<15 mm Hg), then a fluid bolus should be administered. If the wedge pressure is greater than 18 mm Hg, then inotropes are titrated to produce a mixed venous saturation of greater than 70% and a normal lactate level [75].

In studies of traumatic head injuries, the intermittent jugular bulb oxygen saturation monitoring did not significantly influence the management of severe head trauma. Its routine use in all patients seems inadvisable [76].

Hip fractures

Osteoporosis and tendency to fall increase the incidence of hip fractures, which is the most common cause of traumatic injury in geriatric patients, mainly in women. Hip fracture can occur as part of a multitrauma or as an isolated injury. Multitrama is associated with other bone and soft-tissue injuries, intra-abdominal and intrapelvic injuries, major blood loss, head and neck injuries, and other extremity injuries. Overall, an inability to return to a preinjury level of mobility results in precipitous functional decline, a loss of independence, quality of life reduction, and depression in older persons. There are data to suggest that outcome in these patients is superior when they are managed by a specialized multidisciplinary team [77].

Most data indicate that early operation is coupled with improved prognosis and enhanced health quality, even at the same day of injury [78]. Recent data suggest a 48-hour window to operate on patients [79,80]. Delaying surgery may increase mortality [81] or prolong hospitalization [82].

Early ambulation and daily physical therapy after hip fracture surgery should be encouraged. Delayed ambulation after hip fracture surgery is related to the development of new-onset delirium, postoperative pneumonia, and increased length of hospital stay [83].

There are no conclusive data concerning the advantage of regional versus general anesthetic techniques to facilitate surgery for a broken hip. Outcome studies have failed to show a difference between the techniques [84]. No difference has been shown in inpatient morbidity and mortality or in 1-year mortality rates between patients receiving general or spinal anesthesia. There is no significant difference in postoperative cognitive functioning between the two techniques [85]. In addition, comparing regional and general anesthesia, no differences were observed in long-term recovery of ambulatory ability or percent functional recovery after hip fracture [86,87]. This lack of difference has been reflected by a large meta-analysis looking at the elderly surgical population [88].

Head injuries

Elderly persons are at high risk for traumatic brain injury [49]. However, much of the evidence suffers from severe methodologic flaws. Our understanding of the management of such injuries has been improving steadily [89]. The adverse impact of serious head injury on early and delayed mortality has been reported [4,90]. Falls are the most common cause of head injuries in the elderly population, followed by pedestrian injuries [91]. There is a high incidence of intracranial bleeding associated with falls in elderly patients [92].

Age seems to be an independent predictor of poor outcome in patients with head injury [93]. There seems to be an increased mortality in older patients [94]. It has been reported that the mortality of patients with severe brain injury was around 38% for all age groups; however, among persons over 55 years of age, mortality is 80% [95].

A low score on the Glasgow Coma Scale (GCS) is associated with poor outcome in the elderly population [96]. The literature does not identify a specific admission GCS as being applicable as a basis for triage of such patients.

Alteration in orientation possibly points to injury of the central nervous system. Increased vascular vulnerability is characteristic of the aging brain. Subdural hematomas can result in changes in mental status, headache, disturbances in ambulation, or nonfocal neurologic findings. Elderly patients frequently suffer from coexisting medical problems and may take medications, such as anticoagulants, that could worsen head injuries [97].

A baseline level of consciousness should be ascertained. The GCS is a useful tool for such evaluation. Changes from the initial GCS score are important in following clinical progress. It seems reasonable to conclude that initial assertive treatment is warranted in all geriatric patients who have head injuries. Patients who do not respond to such efforts in a timely fashion probably will have poor outcomes, and continuation of such aggressive approaches should be reconsidered. The prognosis is favorable for those who respond to such initial intense efforts.

Many techniques of intubation and choices of drugs exist for safe endotracheal intubation of the patient who has traumatic brain injury. The best technique is the one performed by a proficient anesthesiologist. Oral intubation using direct laryngoscopy facilitated by intravenous induction agents and neuromuscular relaxants is the method of choice [98]. Cricoid pressure is used to prevent passive gastric regurgitation; however, it has been postulated that the application of cricoid pressure may aggravate potential cervical spine injuries [99]. Therefore, the risk of gastric regurgitation should be weighed against the chance of cervical injury when contemplating the Selick maneuver. The elderly population has a greater incidence of cervical spinal disease, which probably increases the risk of instability [100].

Sodium thiopental, etomidate hydrochloride, and propofol have been used to induce anesthesia before intubation. No single agent has been shown to be superior. Each decreases the systemic response to intubation, blunts Intracranial Pressure (ICP) changes, and decreases the cerebral metabolic rate for oxygen [101].

Inadequate fluid resuscitation is associated with poor neurologic outcome in patients who have head injury [102]. On the other hand, fluid overload should be avoided among elderly patients who have concurrent cardiac disease. It has been suggested that patients who have diffuse blunt trauma and closed-head injuries have evidence of impaired peripheral perfusion. This is true even when they are normotensive. In such patients, volume infusion and vasodilating inotropic support improve oxygen transport without increasing intracranial pressure [103].

Summary

Modern society is characterized as having an ever enlarging population of older adults. There are more elderly patients, and the average age of this group is increasing. The anesthetic management of surgery for the elderly trauma victim is more complicated than in younger adults. Evaluation of the physiologic status of the geriatric patient should take into account the variability of the changes associated with advancing age. These alterations occur between individuals and among different organ systems within an individual. In addition, changes in the occurrence and presentation of certain diseases differ. This increases the likelihood of multiple medical diagnoses and is the basis of reduced functional reserve.

A number of elderly persons are independent and have preserved lean body mass and cardiopulmonary function. They have physiologic responses similar to those of younger individuals. In these patients, the risks associated with surgical intervention are low. Conversely, elderly persons who have multiple illnesses and limited capacity suffer from cardiovascular and pulmonary disease and have high surgery-associated risks.

Because of these confounding variables, the potential benefits and the risks of any intervention are more difficult to assess in older persons. Making assumptions about physiologic status that are reasonable in younger patients may not be appropriate in older patients. Occasionally, in clearly identified patients, an early aggressive approach may prevent morbidity.

Several factors are critical for obtaining the best outcomes for the perioperative management of the elderly trauma patient:(1) careful preoperative evaluation and optimization; (2) minimization of perioperative stresses of hypothermia, hypoxemia, and pain; and (3) meticulous perioperative attention to avoid clinical complications from fluid and electrolyte balance and impaired cardiovascular and respiratory function. Care of the injured elderly patient requires thorough preoperative assessment and planning and the involvement of a multidisciplinary clinical team knowledgeable about and interested in the management of the elderly surgical patient [104]. With such an inclusive methodology, major surgeries can be tackled with low risk, a brief hospital stay, and a rapid return to full function as the goal of care [105].

References

[1] Max W, Rice DP, MacKenzie EJ. The lifetime cost of injury. Injury 1990;27:332–43.
[2] Sjogren H, Bjornstig U. Trauma in the elderly: the impact on the health care system. Scand J Prim Health Care 1991;9:203–7.
[3] Testa JA, Malec JF, Moessner AM, et al. Outcome after traumatic brain injury: effects of aging on recovery. Arch Phys Med Rehabil 2005;86:1815–23.
[4] McMahon DJ, Schwab CW, Kauder D. Comorbidity and the elderly trauma patient. World J Surg 1996;20:1113–9.
[5] Travis KW, Mihevc NT, Orkin FK, et al. Age and anesthetic practice: a regional perspective. J Clin Anesth 1999;11:175–186.
[6] Sklar DP, Demarest GB, McFeeley P. Increased pedestrian mortality among the elderly. Am J Emerg Med 1989;7:387–90.
[7] Johnson CL, Margulies DR, Kearney TJ, et al. Trauma in the elderly: an analysis of outcomes based on age. Am Surg 1994;60:899–902.

[8] Muhlberg W, Platt D. Age-dependent changes of the kidneys: pharmacological implications. Gerontology 1999;45:243–53.

[9] Buemi M, Nostro L, Aloisi C, et al. Kidney aging: from phenotype to genetics. Rejuvenation Res 2005;8:101–9.

[10] Janssens JP. Aging of the respiratory system: impact on pulmonary function tests and adaptation to exertion. Clin Chest Med 2005;26:469–84.

[11] Williams JM, Evans TC. Acute pulmonary disease in the aged. Clin Geriatr Med 1993;9: 527–45.

[12] Cardus J, Burgos F, Diaz O, et al. Increase in pulmonary ventilation-perfusion inequality with age in healthy individuals. Am J Respir Crit Care Med 1997;156:648–53.

[13] Nickalls RW, Mapleson WW. Age-related iso-MAC charts for isoflurane, sevoflurane and desflurane in man. Br J Anaesth 2003;91:170–4.

[14] Thompson LF. Failure to wean: exploring the influence of age-related pulmonary changes. Crit Care Nurs Clin North Am 1996;8:7–16.

[15] Chalfin DB. Outcome assessment in elderly patients with critical illness and respiratory failure. ClinChest Med 1993;14:583–9.

[16] Mooradian AD. Normal age-related changes in thyroid hormone economy. Clin Geriatr Med 1995;11:159–69.

[17] Barton RN, Horan MA, Clague JE, et al. The effect of aging on the metabolic clearance rate and distribution of cortisol in man. Arch Gerontol Geriatr 1999;29:95–105.

[18] Frankenfield D, Cooney RN, Smith JS, et al. Age-related differences in the metabolic response to injury. J Trauma 2000;48:49–56.

[19] Demarest GB, Osler TM, Clevenger FW. Injuries in the elderly: evaluation and initial response. Geriatrics 1990;45:36–8, 41–2.

[20] Scwab C, Shapiro M, Kauder D. Geriatric trauma: patterns, care and outcomes. In: Mattox K, Feliciano D, Moore E, editors. Trauma. New York: McGraw-Hill; 2000. p. 1099–113.

[21] Lane P, Sorondo B, Kelly JJ. Geriatric trauma patients-are they receiving trauma center care? Acad Emerg Med 2003;10:244–50.

[22] McKinley BA, Marvin RG, Cocanour CS, et al. Blunt trauma resuscitation: the old can respond. Arch Surg 2000;135:688–93.

[23] Gubler KD, Davis R, Koepsell T, et al. Long-term survival of elderly trauma patients. Arch Surg 1997;132:1010–4.

[24] DeMaria EJ, Kenney PR, Merriam MA, et al. Aggressive trauma care benefits the elderly. J Trauma 1987;27:1200–6.

[25] Shabot MM, Johnson CL. Outcome from critical care in the "oldest old" trauma patients. J Trauma 1995;39:254–9.

[26] Yee WY, Cameron PA, Bailey MJ. Road traffic injuries in the elderly. Emerg Med J 2006; 23:42–6.

[27] McCoy GF, Johnstone RA, Duthie RB. Injury to the elderly in road traffic accidents. J Trauma 1989;29:494–7.

[28] Allen JE, Schwab CW. Blunt chest trauma in the elderly. Am Surg 1985;51:697–700.

[29] Riggs BL, Melton LJ 3rd. Involutional osteoporosis. N Engl J Med 1986;26(314):1676–86.

[30] Morris JA Jr, MacKenzie EJ, Edelstein SL. The effect of preexisting conditions on mortality in trauma patients. JAMA 1990;11(263):1942–6.

[31] Pudelek B. Geriatric trauma: special needs for a special population. AACN Clin Issues 2002;13:61–72.

[32] Wofford JL, Moran WP, Heuser MD, et al. Emergency medical transport of the elderly: a population-based study. Am J Emerg Med 1995;13:297–300.

[33] McMahon DJ, Shapiro MB, Kauder DR. The injured elderly in the trauma intensive care unit. Surg Clin North Am 2000;80:1005–19.

[34] Hurst JM, DeHaven CB, Branson RD. Use of CPAP mask as the sole mode of ventilatory support in trauma patients with mild to moderate respiratory insufficiency. J Trauma 1985; 25:1065–8.

[35] Mosenthal AC, Livingston DH, Elcavage J, et al. Epidemiology and strategies for prevention. J Trauma 1995;38:753–6.

[36] Velmahos GC, Jindal A, Chan LS. "Insignificant" mechanism of injury: not to be taken lightly. J Am Coll Surg 2001;192:147–52.

[37] Lambert DA, Sattin RW. Death from falls, 1978-1984. MMWR 1998;37(SS-1):21–6.

[38] Ruhle R, Wolff H. Psychological aspects of traffic fitness of aging car drivers. Z Gesamte Hyg 1990;3:346–50.

[39] Sjogren H, Eriksson A, Ostrom M. Role of disease in initiating the crashes of fatally injured drivers. Accid Anal Prev 1996;28:307–14.

[40] Linn BS. Age differences in the severity and outcome of burns. J Am Geriatr Soc 1980;28: 118–23.

[41] Kennedy RD. Elder abuse and neglect: the experience, knowledge, and attitudes of primary care physicians. Fam Med 2005;37:481–5.

[42] Elder abuse and neglect. Council on Scientific Affairs. JAMA 1987;257:966–71.

[43] Finelli FC, Jonsson J, Champion HR, et al. A case control study for major trauma in geriatric patients. J Trauma 1989;29:541–8.

[44] Phillips S, Rond PC III, Kelly SM, et al. The failure of triage criteria to identify geriatric patients with trauma: results from the Florida Trauma Triage Study. J Trauma 1996;40:278–83.

[45] Scheetz LJ. Relationship of age, injury severity, injury type, comorbid conditions, level of care, and survival among older motor vehicle trauma patients. Res Nurs Health 2005;28: 198–209.

[46] Perdue PW, Watts DD, Kaufmann CR, et al. Differences in mortality between elderly and younger adult trauma patients: geriatric status increases risk of delayed death. J Trauma 1998;45:805–10.

[47] Knudson MM, Lieberman J, Morris JA Jr, et al. Mortality factors in geriatric blunt trauma patients. Arch Surg 1994;129:448–53.

[48] Davis JW, Kaups KL. Base deficit in the elderly: a marker of severe injury and death. J Trauma 1998;45:873–7.

[49] Tieves KS, Yang H, Layde PM. The epidemiology of traumatic brain injury in Wisconsin, 2001. WMJ 2005;104:22–5, 54.

[50] Martyn JA, White DA, Gronert GA, et al. Up and down regulation of skeletal muscle acetylcholine receptors. Anesthesiology 1992;76:822–43.

[51] Tornetta P III, Mostafavi H, Riina J, et al. Morbidity and mortality in elderly trauma patients. J Trauma 1999;46:702–6.

[52] Adnet F, Lapostolle F, Ricard-Hibon A, et al. Intubating trauma patients before reaching hospital—revisited. Crit Care 2001;5:290–1.

[53] Berkenstadt H, Mayan H, Segal E, et al. The pharmacokinetics of morphine and lidocaine in nine severe trauma patients. J Clin Anesth 1999;11:630–4.

[54] Eilers H, Niemann C. Clinically important drug interactions with intravenous anaesthetics in older patients. Drugs Aging 2003;20:969–80.

[55] Vuyk J. Pharmacodynamics in the elderly. Best Pract Res Clin Anaesthesiol 2003;17: 207–18.

[56] Arden JR, Holley FO, Stanski DR. Increased sensitivity to etomidate in the elderly: initial distribution versus altered brain response. Anesthesiology 1986;65:19–27.

[57] Homer TD, Stanski DR. The effect of increasing age on thiopental disposition and anesthetic requirement. Anesthesiology 1985;62:714–24.

[58] Reves JG, Fragen RJ, Vinik HR, et al. Midazolam: pharmacology and uses. Anesthesiology 1985;62:310–24.

[59] Smith MR, Bell GD, Quine MA, et al. Small bolus injections of intravenous midazolam for upper gastrointestinal endoscopy: a study of 788 consecutive cases. Br J Clin Pharmacol 1993;36:573–8.

[60] Kaiko RF, Wallenstein SL, Rogers AG, et al. Narcotics in the elderly. Med Clin North Am 1982;66:1079–89.

[61] Shafer SL. The pharmacology of anesthetic drugs in the elderly patients. Anesthesiol Clin North America 2000;18:1–29.

[62] Minto CF, Schnider TW, Egan TD, et al. Influence of age and gender on the pharmacokinetics and pharmacodynamics of remifentanil: I. Model development. Anesthesiology 1997;86:10–23.

[63] Herman RJ, McAllister CB, Branch RA, et al. Effects of age on meperidine disposition. Clin Pharmacol Ther 1985;37:19–24.

[64] Rupp SM, Castagnoli KP, Fisher DM, et al. Pancuronium and vecuronium pharmacokinetics and pharmacodynamics in younger and elderly adults. Anesthesiology 1987;67:45–9.

[65] Milzman DP, Rothenhaus TC. Resuscitation of the geriatric patient. Emerg Med Clin North Am 1996;14:233–44.

[66] Pontoppidan H, Beecher HK. Progressive loss of protective reflexes in the airway with the advance of age. JAMA 1960;174:2209–13.

[67] Givol N, Gershtansky Y, Halamish-Shani T, et al. Perianesthetic dental injuries: analysis of incident reports. J Clin Anesth 2004;16:173–6.

[68] Benumof JL. Management of the difficult adult airway: with special emphasis on awake tracheal intubation. Anesthesiology 1991;75:1087–110.

[69] Scalea TM, Simon HM, Duncan AO, et al. Geriatric blunt multiple trauma: improved survival with early invasive monitoring. J Trauma 1990;30:129–34.

[70] Santora TA, Schinco MA, Trooskin SZ. Management of trauma in the elderly patient. Surg Clin North Am 1994;74:163–86.

[71] Hiatt JR, Yeatman LA Jr, Child JS. The value of echocardiography in blunt chest trauma. J Trauma 1988;28:914–22.

[72] Guryel E, Redfern DJ, Ricketts DM. Balancing priorities in the management of hip fractures: guidelines versus resources. Ann R Coll Surg Engl 2004;86:171–3.

[73] Brown CV, Shoemaker WC, Wo CC, et al. Is noninvasive hemodynamic monitoring appropriate for the elderly critically injured patient? J Trauma 2005;58:102–7.

[74] Venn R, Steele A, Richardson P, et al. Randomized controlled trial to investigate influence of the fluid challenge on duration of hospital stay and perioperative morbidity in patients with hip fractures. Br J Anaesth 2002;88:65–71.

[75] Shoemaker WC. Oxygen transport and oxygen metabolism in shock and critical illness: invasive and noninvasive monitoring of circulatory dysfunction and shock. Crit Care Clin 1996;12:939–69.

[76] Latronico N, Beindorf AE, Rasulo FA, et al. Limits of intermittent jugular bulb oxygen saturation monitoring in the management of severe head trauma patients. Neurosurgery 2001;48:454–6.

[77] Khasraghi FA, Christmas C, Lee EJ, et al. Effectiveness of a multidisciplinary team approach to hip fracture management. J Surg Orthop Adv 2005;14:27–31.

[78] Casaletto JA, Gatt R. Post-operative mortality related to waiting time for hip fracture surgery. Injury 2004;35:114–20.

[79] Doruk H, Mas MR, Yildiz C, et al. The effect of the timing of hip fracture surgery on the activity of daily living and mortality in elderly. Arch Gerontol Geriatr 2004;39:179–85.

[80] Gdalevich M, Cohen D, Yosef D, et al. Morbidity and mortality after hip fracture: the impact of operative delay. Arch Orthop Trauma Surg 2004;124:334–40.

[81] Moran CG, Wenn RT, Sikand M, et al. Early mortality after hip fracture: is delay before surgery important? J Bone Joint Surg Am 2005;87:483–9.

[82] Siegmeth AW, Gurusamy K, Parker MJ. Delay to surgery prolongs hospital stay in patients with fractures of the proximal femur. J Bone Joint Surg Br 2005;87:1123–6.

[83] Kamel HK, Iqbal MA, Mogallapu R, et al. Time to ambulation after hip fracture surgery: relation to hospitalization outcomes. J Gerontol A Biol Sci Med Sci 2003;58:1042–5.

[84] O'Hara DA, Duff A, Berlin JA, et al. The effect of anesthetic technique on postoperative outcomes in hip fracture repair. Anesthesiology 2000;92:928–30.

[85] Berggren D, Gustafson Y, Eriksson B, et al. Postoperative confusion after anesthesia in elderly patients with femoral neck fractures. Anesth Analg 1987;66:497–504.

[86] Koval KJ, Aharonoff GB, Rosenberg AD, et al. Functional outcome after hip fracture: effect of general versus regional anesthesia. Clin Orthop Relat Res 1998;348:37–41.

[87] Gilbert TB, Hawkes WG, Hebel JR, et al. Spinal anesthesia versus general anesthesia for hip fracture repair: a longitudinal observation of 741 elderly patients during 2-year follow-up. Am J Orthop 2000;29:25–35.

[88] Parker MJ, Handoll HH, Griffiths R. Anaesthesia for hip fracture surgery in adults. Cochrane Database Syst Rev 2001;18:CD000521.

[89] Lillehei KO, Hoff JT. Advances in the management of closed head injury. Ann Emerg Med 1985;14:789–95.

[90] Champion HR, Copes WS, Buyer D, et al. Major trauma in geriatric patients. Am J Public Health 1989;79:1278–82.

[91] Pentland B, Hutton LS, Jones PA. Late mortality after head injury. J Neurol Neurosurg Psychiatry 2005;76:395–400.

[92] Amacher AL, Bybee DE. Toleration of head injury by the elderly. Neurosurgery 1987;20: 954–8.

[93] Mosenthal AC, Livingston DH, Lavery RF, et al. The effect of age on functional outcome in mild traumatic brain injury: 6-month report of a prospective multicenter trial. J Trauma 2004;56:1042–8.

[94] Mosenthal AC, Lavery RF, Addis M, et al. Isolated traumatic brain injury: age is an independent predictor of mortality and early outcome. J Trauma 2002;52:907–11.

[95] Vollmer DG. Age and outcome following traumatic coma: why do older patients fare worse? Neurosurg 1991;75:S37–49.

[96] Reuter F. Traumatic intracranial hemorrhages in elderly people. Adv Neurosurg 1989;17: 43–8.

[97] Lehman LB. Head trauma in the elderly. Postgrad Med 1988;82:140–2.

[98] Alker GJ, Oh YS, Leslie EV, et al. Postmortem radiology of head and neck injuries in fatal traffic accidents. Radiology 1975;114:611–7.

[99] Donaldson WF 3rd, Towers JD, Doctor A, et al. A methodology to evaluate motion of the unstable spine during intubation techniques. Spine 1993;18:2020–3.

[100] Irvine DH, Foster JB, Newell DJ. Prevalence of cervical spondylosis in a general practice. Lancet 1965;22(14):1089–92.

[101] Unni VKN, Johnston RA, Young HSA, et al. Prevention of intracranial hypertension during laryngoscopy and endotracheal intubation. Br J Anaesth 1984;56:1219–23.

[102] Clifton GL, Miller ER, Choi SC, et al. Fluid thresholds and outcome from severe brain injury. Crit Care Med 2002;30:739–45.

[103] Scalea TM, Maltz S, Yelon J, et al. Resuscitation of multiple trauma and head injury: role of crystalloid fluids and inotropes. Crit Care Med 1994;22:1610–5.

[104] Callum K, Gray A, Hoile R, et al. Extremes of age. 1999 NCEPOD report. London: National Confidential Enquiry into Perioperative Deaths; 1999.

[105] Bardram L, Funch-Jensen P, Kehlet H. Rapid rehabilitation in elderly patients after laparoscopic colonic resection. Br J Surg 2000;87:1540–5.

ELSEVIER
SAUNDERS

Anesthesiology Clin
25 (2007) 91–98

ANESTHESIOLOGY
CLINICS

Management of the Obese Trauma Patient

Yuval Meroz, MD, Yaacov Gozal, MD*

*Department of Anesthesiology & CCM, Hadassah Hebrew University
School of Medicine, Hadassah Medical Organization, Kiryat Hadassah,
P.O. Box 12000, Jerusalem 91120, Israel*

Trauma and obesity are large-scale epidemics, causing significant morbidity and mortality. About 35% of Americans are overweight, with a body mass index (BMI) of 25 to 29 kg/m^2; about 25% are obese (BMI of 30–39); and 5% are morbidly obese (BMI $\geq$ 40) [1]. This increasing population of overweight and morbidly obese persons will undoubtedly cause an increasing population of obese trauma victims. Despite the abundance of studies about trauma and morbid obesity, there are few studies about the impact of morbid obesity on type of injury, complications, and outcome. Thus, the aim of this article is to review the literature about the following subjects:

Are obese patients at a higher risk for trauma?
Do they suffer different types of injury?
Are they more prone to complications after injury?
Should treatment be modified when obese trauma victims are involved?

Before the trauma: risk of injury

Obesity has been found to be associated with a higher rate of overall injuries among children [2] and adults [3]. Obesity's effect on serious injuries, especially motor vehicle accidents, is less clear. Sleep apnea is a proven risk factor for vehicle accidents. Findley and colleagues [4] found that persons with sleep apnea had a sevenfold risk for vehicle accidents, compared with persons without sleep apnea. Teran-Santos and colleagues [5] performed a sleep test on 102 drivers who were involved in traffic accidents

---

* Corresponding author.
E-mail address: gozaly@md.huji.ac.il (Y. Gozal).

0889-8537/07/$ - see front matter © 2007 Elsevier Inc. All rights reserved.
doi:10.1016/j.atc.2006.11.005
anesthesiology.theclinics.com

and compared the results to those of 152 matched controls. They found that persons with significant sleep apnea had an odds ratio of 6.3 of being involved in a traffic accident. Although sleep apnea is not a synonym for obesity, there is a very strong correlation between both diseases. About 70% of sleep apnea patients are obese and about 40% of obese persons suffer from sleep apnea [6,7]. In a cohort study from New Zealand, Whitlock and colleagues [8] investigated the association between driver's risk of injury and BMI. This half-prospective and half-retrospective study included 10,525 persons whose records were analyzed for a mean follow-up period of 10.3 years. Obesity (BMI $\geq$ 28.7) was associated with a twofold risk for injury in a traffic accident, even after adjustment for other variables.

Prehospital: type of injury

Several works have evaluated the difference in injury patterns between obese and nonobese patients. The question about different types of injury arises not only because of different body habitus, but also because vehicles are designed to fit and provide safety to passengers with an average height and weight. In 1992, Boulanger and colleagues [9] analyzed the data on 6368 adults admitted to a level 1 trauma center because of blunt trauma over a 4-year period. They found that obese victims (BMI > 31) had significantly more rib fractures, pulmonary contusions, pelvic fractures, and extremity fractures, and fewer head and liver injuries. Moran and colleagues [10] searched the National Automotive Sampling System Crashworthiness Data System from 1995 to 1999. Their hypothesis was that if a driver's body habitus diverges from the 50% percentile male Hybrid III Crash Dummy, the pattern of injury changes. Their results showed similar results to those of Boulanger and colleagues [9], with significantly fewer head and abdominal injury in patients with a BMI higher than 31. Another large retrospective study, by Mock and colleagues [11], based on the National Automotive Sampling System data from 1993 to 1996, showed increased risk of chest injuries among overweight vehicle crash victims. In a relatively small prospective work, Arbabi and colleagues [12] analyzed the data of 189 patients over 13 years old who were injured at a motor vehicle crash and transported to a level 1 trauma center. They found that overweight (BMI of 25–30) victims had a lower Injury Severity Score (ISS), increased severity of lower extremity injuries, and reduced severity of abdominal injuries. Obese patients (BMI > 30) also suffered a greater severity of lower extremity injury, but their ISS and abdominal injury severity were comparable to their lean counterparts, and there was no difference regarding head injury.

The importance of this work was the introduction of the "cushion effect" hypothesis. The cushion effect is the increased protection given by the thicker abdominal fat layer of obese people to the internal organs, therefore reducing abdominal injuries. The cushion effect can protect overweight but not obese patients, because obese patients' high mass and kinetic energy can overwhelm the protective effect of the abdominal fat. It is unclear if this cushion effect is effective in other types of trauma besides vehicle crashes. A larger, but retrospective, study was done by Byrens and colleagues [13], who analyzed the files of 1877 adult patients admitted to a level 1 trauma center during 1 year. Only 1179 patients were included because of a lack of data. This large study did not show any difference in injury patterns between patients with a BMI higher than 35 and those with a BMI less than 35. Some conflicting results came from another large retrospective study by Brown and colleagues [14] that included 1153 patients, all of whom suffered blunt trauma that required admission to an ICU at a level 1 trauma center. Patients were classified as obese (BMI $\geq$ 30) or nonobese (BMI < 30). Obese patients had significantly fewer head injuries (42% versus 55%), but suffered significantly more lower extremity fractures (53% versus 38%). Recently, this group examined the impact of obesity on children and adolescents [15]. Obese patients (BMI $\geq$ 95th percentile for age) suffered significantly fewer severe head injuries (20% AIS $\geq$ 3) than nonobese patients (38%), despite similar ISS for both groups. The results showed a tendency toward fewer overall head injuries, but without statistical significance.

In summary, obese patients tend to have fewer head injuries and more lower extremity, pelvic, and rib fractures. Overweight, but not obese, patients involved in motor vehicle accidents may have some abdominal protective or cushion effect. However, these findings should not justify a different approach to obese patients at the prehospital stage or at the emergency room. The findings should be considered, however, when designing safety devices to give obese persons an adequate level of protection that is comparable to that given to their lean counterparts.

In hospital: complications, morbidity, and mortality

Overweight patients are prone to develop more complications following trauma than lean patients. The first work to show a worse outcome in overweight patients was the study by Choban and colleagues [16] in 1991. This retrospective work analyzed the charts of 351 patients suffering blunt trauma. Unfortunately, only 184 records had height and weight data. The main findings showed significantly high mortality rates (42.1% for the severely overweight group [BMI > 31], compared with 8.0% for the overweight group [BMI of 27–31], and 5.0% for the average weight group [BMI < 27]). The severely overweight patients suffered more complications, mainly pulmonary in nature. The clinical course of the severely overweight nonsurvivors was characterized by a significantly shorter length of stay at hospital (8.62 days versus 26.6 days for the average weight group) and a rapid deterioration, unresponsive to intervention. Increased BMI and ISS were found to be independent determinants of outcome. Mock and colleagues [11] found that increased weight and a higher BMI were strong predictors of 30-days mortality. The odds ratios of risk of death were 2.57 for a body weight of 100 to 119 kg, and 4.48 for a body weight above 119 kg. For increased BMI, the odds ratios were 3.18 for a BMI of 35 to 39 and 3.34 for a BMI above 39, all statistically significant. The investigators speculated that increased mortality could be attributed at least partially to a higher rate of comorbidities among the obese patients. Increased body weight and increased BMI remained associated with increased mortality after a multivariate logistic regression analysis that included adjustment for age, gender, seatbelt use, seating position, and vehicle weight.

Arbabi and colleagues [12] found that for the lean patients, the mean ISS was 26.3 and the mortality rate was 11.3%. For the overweight patients, the mean ISS was 19.4 and the mortality rate was 4.9%. The mean ISS of the obese patients was 23.1, similar to the ISS of their lean counterparts, but the mortality rate was significantly higher (20% versus 11.3%, OR = 4.2). Therefore, the increased mortality rate appears to be related to the increased BMI, and not to severity of injury. The nonlinear association (reduced mortality rate for overweight patients compared with either lean or obese patients) probably was caused by the cushion effect described previously.

Wang and colleagues [17] analyzed the data of 67 patients who were involved in motor vehicle collisions and underwent abdominal CT. Increased depth of subcutaneous fat was associated with decreased severity of abdominal injury. The influence of the victim's gender was not examined until Zhu and colleagues [18] analyzed National Automotive Sampling System data between the years 1997 and 2001. A total of 30,667 victims were enrolled, of whom 8230 were excluded. The end point was 30-days mortality. Although men had a nonlinear J-shaped association between their BMI and mortality, with lowest risk at a BMI of 28, women's' risk had no association with their BMI. Additionally, women with elevated BMIs had a lower risk, compared with men with elevated BMIs. The pattern of the men can be explained by the cushion effect, but the pattern of the women is unclear and might be associated with different body shape or different distribution of subcutaneous fat. Byrens and colleagues [13] found that the overall mortality rate of obese (BMI $\geq$ 35) patients was 10.7%, compared with 4.1% for patients with a BMI of less than 35. The mortality rate of obese patients with an ISS of at least 20 was 56.3%, compared with 20.2% for nonobese patients. The rate of complications was also significantly higher. Generally, 27% of the obese patients had at least one complication, compared with 17.6% of the lean patients. More specifically, obese patients had more pulmonary complications, such as adult respiratory distress syndrome, found in 6.5% of the obese group versus 2% of the lean patients, and the need for mechanical ventilation (14.7% of obese patients versus 9% of lean patients). These findings cannot be explained by pre-existing diseases only, because both groups had a similar percentage of chronic obstructive pulmonary disease. The obese patients also suffered a higher rate of renal complications, including acute renal failure and acute renal insufficiency (6.6% of the obese patients versus 1% of the lean patients). Twenty-five percent of the obese patients with an ISS of at least 20 developed renal complications, compared with 2.2% of their lean counterparts. Obese patients had significantly higher rates of diabetes and hypertension, which could partially explain the high percentage of renal complications. On the other hand, the rate of cardiovascular complications was similar between the groups.

One of the main results of this study is the definition of a BMI of greater than or equal to 35 as a cutoff point for increased risk for trauma victims. In a retrospective study of 242 blunt trauma victims admitted to a level 1 trauma center, Neville and colleagues [19] showed that patients with a BMI of greater than or equal to 30 suffered a twofold increase in mortality compared with lean patients (32% versus 16%) and a fourfold increase in the rate of multiple organ failure (13% versus 3%). In the work of Brown and colleagues [14], obesity was found to be an independent risk factor for mortality (odds ratio = 1.6). Obese patients suffered more overall complications (42% versus 32%), more multiple system organ failure (19% versus 11%), more adult respiratory distress syndrome (11% versus 6%), and more renal failure requiring dialysis (8% versus 4%). In a short publication, Zein and colleagues [20] described 304 patients admitted to an ICU at a level 1 trauma center. Most of the patients were men (75%) and suffered blunt trauma (86%). Obese patients made up 33% of the study population and suffered an overall mortality rate of 11.3%, similar to the 12.1% rate of the nonobese patients. These findings contradict other published works. Brown and colleagues [15] examined the effect of obesity on children suffering trauma. The study included 316 patients, aged 6 to19, who were treated in an ICU in a level 1 trauma center. Patients were classified as obese (BMI $\geq$ 9th percentile for age) or nonobese. The mortality rates were not statistically different between the obese (9%) and nonobese (15%) children.

It seems that morbid obesity is an independent risk factor for mortality following severe trauma, and the risk may be a two- to fourfold increase. Obese patients suffer many more pulmonary and renal complications, with an increased need for prolonged mechanical ventilation. Patients of moderate weight, with a BMI of around 28, seem to have some protection, compared with lean and obese patients, and these patients are less prone to mortality and complications. The studies are mostly retrospective, and many patients, up to 50%, were omitted because of a lack of data. Some works included only vehicle crash victims, whereas others included all blunt trauma victims, or even penetrating trauma victims. The common BMI definitions for obesity might not be adequate for trauma patients. At least one large study suggests that the cutoff limit for increased risk should be a BMI higher than 35. As to specific treatment or approach, the authors recommend using increased BMI as a risk factor, especially while considering admission to an ICU.

Treating the obese trauma patient: clinical topics

Because of the lack of studies and guidelines about the clinical approach to the obese trauma patient, it is necessary to rely on either small series and case reports or general articles about treating obese critical patients [21–24]. Securing the airway is the first priority. Using gum elastic bougie has been recommended for cases of difficult intubation [25], and the laryngeal mask [26] or Combitube [27] can be used as a rescue device. A combination of rigid laryngoscopy and fiberoptic bronchoscope can be used for tube exchanging [28], but fiberoptic intubation can be limited by the presence of blood and secretions. Securing the surgical airway can be challenging as well. Even after a period of time in the ICU, conversion from endotracheal tube to tracheostomy might be difficult. Rehm and colleagues [29] studied cases in which elective cricothyroidotomy was performed instead of tracheostomy in 18 morbidly obese trauma patients after prolonged intubation in the ICU. None of the patients suffered any major complications related to the procedure and the investigators found that cricothyroidotomy can be a reasonable and less demanding alternative to tracheostomy in ventilated patients with difficult neck anatomy. Weaning the injured obese patient might be challenging as well. Yoo and colleagues [30] reported their experience with a 69-year-old obese patient (BMI = 39) suffering multiple rib fractures and pulmonary contusion. Weaning was successful only after abdominal lipectomy and omentectomy, with removal of 4.5 kg of abdominal fat.

Another important issue in treating obese trauma patients is the risk of thromboembolic events. Both trauma and obesity are independent risk factors for such events [31]. Meissner and colleagues [32] conducted a prospective study that included 101 trauma patients with ISS greater than or equal to 15. Obesity, defined as a body weight higher than 120% of ideal body weight among men and higher than 130% among women, was found to be an independent risk factor for thromboembolic events. Although only 4.2% of the patients without venous thromboembolism were obese, as many as 26.7% of the patients suffering venous thromboembolism were obese. Rutherford and colleagues [33] studied the levels of anti-Xa in 18 critically ill trauma and surgical patients, both obese and nonobese. They found that a daily dose of enoxaparin, 40 mg, resulted in an inadequate level of anti-Xa in all but two patients. The investigators' recommendation was a twice-daily regimen and the monitoring of anti-Xa in patients with either morbid obesity or renal failure.

An essential part of treating trauma patients is metabolic and nutritional support, but hemodynamic monitoring can be challenging in obese trauma victims. Line placement can be technically difficult, and the standard equipment may be inadequate. Thompson and colleagues [34] reported a case of extravasation into subcutaneous tissues because the introducer of the pulmonary artery catheter was too short. Brown and colleagues [35] checked the usefulness of cardiac index measurement by thoracic bioimpedance. They compared thermodilution and bioimpedance measurements in 74 obese patients and 211 nonobese patients. All patients were trauma victims admitted to an ICU in a level 1 trauma center. The investigators found the bioimpedance results correlated well with thermodilution measurements in both groups.

Summary

Obese persons are more likely to be involved in vehicle accidents, probably because of the presence of sleep apnea. They are more likely to suffer chest, pelvis, and extremity fractures. Mildly overweight persons are less prone to intra-abdominal injury, because of the protective effect of the abdominal fat, known as the cushion effect. Obese trauma patients are far more likely to develop in-hospital complications, especially pulmonary, renal, and thromboembolic complications. The BMI is an independent risk factor for morbidity and mortality after trauma. Because only limited data exist about the correct clinical approach to obese trauma patients, it is necessary to rely on general knowledge about treating obese patients in the ICU. More research is definitely needed to improve the treatment of obese trauma patients.

References

[1] Hedley AA, Ogden CL, Johnson CL, et al. Prevalance of overweight and obesity among US children, adolescents, and adults, 1999–2002. JAMA 2004;291:2847–50.
[2] Bazelmans C, Coppieters Y, Godin I, et al. Is obesity associated with injuries among young people? Eur J Epidemiol 2004;19:1037–42.
[3] Xiang H, Smith GA, Wilkins JR III, et al. Obesity and risk of nonfatal unintentional injuries. Am J Prev Med 2005;29:41–5.
[4] Findley LJ, Unverzagt MF, Suratt PM. Automobile accidents involving patients with obstructive sleep apnea. Am Rev Respir Dis 1988;138:337–40.
[5] Teran-Santos J, Jimenez-Gomez A, Cordero-Guevara J. The association between sleep apnea and the risk of traffic accidents. N Engl J Med 1999;340:847–51.
[6] Young T, Peppard PE, Gottlieb DJ. Epidemiology of obstructive sleep apnea: a population health perspective. Am J Respir Crit Care Med 2002;165:1217–39.
[7] Malthora A, White DP. Obstructive sleep apnoea. Lancet 2002;360:237–45.
[8] Whitlock G, Norton R, Jackson R, et al. Is body mass index a risk factor for motor vehicle driver injury? A cohort study with prospective and retrospective outcomes. Int J Epidemiol 2003;32:147–9.
[9] Boulanger BR, Miltzman D, Mitchell K, et al. Body habitus as a predictor of injury patterns after blunt trauma. J Trauma 1992;33:228–32.
[10] Moran SG, McGwin G, Metzger JS, et al. Injury rates among restrained drivers in motor vehicle collisions: the role of body habitus. J Trauma 2002;52:1116–20.
[11] Mock CN, Grossman DC, Kauffman RP, et al. The relationship between body weight and risk of death and serious injury in motor vehicle crashes. Accid Anal Prev 2002;34:221–8.
[12] Arbabi S, Wahl WL, Hemmila MR, et al. The cushion effect. J Trauma 2003;54:1090–3.
[13] Byrens MC, McDaniel MD, Moore MB, et al. The effect of obesity on outcomes among injured patients. J Trauma 2005;58:232–7.

[14] Brown CVR, Neville AL, Rhee P, et al. The impact of obesity on the outcome of 1,153 critically injured blunt trauma patients. J Trauma 2005;59:1048–51.

[15] Brown CVR, Neville AL, Salim A, et al. The impact of obesity on severely injured children and adolescents. J Pediatr Surg 2006;41:88–91.

[16] Choban PS, Weireter LJ Jr, Maynes C. Obesity and increased mortality in blunt trauma. J Trauma 1991;31:1253–7.

[17] Wang SC, Bednarski B, Patel S, et al. Increased depth of subcutaneous fat is protective against abdominal injuries in motor vehicle collisions. Annu Proc Assoc Adv Automot Med 2003;47:545–9.

[18] Zhu S, Layde PM, Guse CE, et al. Obesity and risk for death due to motor vehicle crashes. Am J Public Health 2006;96:734–9.

[19] Neville AL, Brown CVR, Weng J, et al. Obesity is an independent risk factor of mortality in severely injured blunt trauma patients. Arch Surg 2004;139:983–7.

[20] Zein JG, Albrecht RM, Tawk MM, et al. Effect of obesity on mortality in severely injured blunt trauma patients remains unclear. Arch Surg 2005;140:1130–1.

[21] Flanchbaum L, Choban PS. Surgical implications of obesity. Annu Rev Med 1998;49: 215–34.

[22] Marik P, Varon J. The obese patient in the ICU. Chest 1998;113:492–8.

[23] Grant P, Newcombe M. Emergency management of the morbidly obese. Emerg Med Australas 2004;16:309–17.

[24] Pieracci FM, Barie PS, Pomp A. Critical care of the bariatric patient. Crit Care Med 2006;34: 1796–804.

[25] Jabre P, Combes X, Leroux B. Use of gum elastic bougie for prehospital difficult intubation. Am J Emerg Med 2005;23:552–5.

[26] Aye T, Milne B. Use of the laryngeal mask prior to definitive intubation in a difficult airway: a case report. J Emerg Med 1995;13:711–4.

[27] Agro F, Frass M, Benumof J. The asophageal tracheal combitube as a non-invasive alternative to endotracheal tube. A review. Minerva Anestesiol 2001;67:863–74.

[28] Hagberg CA, Westhofen P. A two-person technique for fiberoptic-aided tracheal extubation/reintubation in intensive care unit (ICU). J Clin Anesth 2003;15:467–70.

[29] Rehm CG, Wanek SM, Gagnon EB, et al. Cricothyroidotomy for elective airway management in critically ill trauma patients with technically challenging neck anatomy. Crit Care 2002;6:531–5.

[30] Yoo KY, Lim SC, Kim YH, et al. Successful weaning from mechanical ventilation after abdominal lipectomy and omentectomy in an obese patient with multiple rib fractures. Br J Anaesth 2006;96:269–70.

[31] Kim V, Spandorfer J. Epidemiology of venous thromboembolic disease. Emerg Med Clin North Am 2001;19:839–59.

[32] Meissner MH, Chandler WL, Elliot JS. Venous thromboembolism in trauma: a local manifestation of systemic hypercoagulability? J Trauma 2003;54:224–31.

[33] Rutherford EJ, Schooler WG, Sredzinski E. Optimal dose of enoxaparin in critically ill trauma and surgical patients. J Trauma 2005;58:1167–70.

[34] Thompson EC, Wilkins HE, Fox VJ, et al. Insufficient length of pulmonary artery introducer in an obese patient. Arch Surg 2004;139:794–6.

[35] Brown CVR, Martin MJ, Shoemaker WC, et al. The effect of obesity on bioimpedance cardiac index. Am J Surg 2005;189:547–51.

ELSEVIER
SAUNDERS

Anesthesiology Clin
25 (2007) 99–116

ANESTHESIOLOGY
CLINICS

Regional Anesthesia in Trauma Patients

Cesare Gregoretti, MD[a],*, Daniela Decaroli, MD[a],
Antonio Miletto, MD[a], Alice Mistretta, MD[b],
Rosario Cusimano, MD[a], V. Marco Ranieri, MD[b]

[a]Dipartimento Emergenza Accettazione, ASO CTO-CRF-Maria Adelaide,
Via Zuretti 29, 10129 Torino, Italy
[b]Università di Torino, Dipartimento di Anestesiologia e Rianimazione,
Ospedale S. Giovanni Battista-Molinette Torino, Corso Bramante 89, 10129 Torino, Italy

Trauma is a major cause of mortality throughout the world and pain is the most common symptom reported by patients admitted to the emergency room [1]. Specific protocols have been developed to treat all pain-related complications, such as posttraumatic stress disorders [2], making anesthesiologists more involved in the management of trauma patients. Even though data demonstrating that regional anesthesia improves outcome are lacking, improved pain management in the trauma patient not only increases comfort and reduces patient suffering but has also been demonstrated to reduce the rate of intubation and morbidity and to improve short- and long-term outcomes [3–6].

Shulz-Stubmer and colleagues [7] reported that regional analgesia using single-injection regional blocks and continuous neuraxial and peripheral catheters can play a valuable role in a multimodal approach to pain management in trauma patients admitted in the intensive care unit.

Although surgical interventions for multiple trauma more frequently require general anesthesia (GA), regional anesthesia (RA) should be considered in patients who have isolated orthopedic injuries [8,9] and in burn patients [7]. A meta-analysis [10] showed that neuraxial blocks significantly reduce postoperative mortality and morbidity (eg, deep vein thrombosis, pulmonary embolism) when compared with general anesthesia, although results for hip fracture repair are still debatable [11].

In this article we (1) describe the use of different techniques of regional anesthesia that could be potentially used in patients who have trauma,

---

* Corresponding author.
E-mail address: c.gregoretti@tiscali.it (C. Gregoretti).

1932-2275/07/$ - see front matter © 2007 Elsevier Inc. All rights reserved.
doi:10.1016/j.anclin.2006.12.002
anesthesiology.theclinics.com

and (2) describe indications, limitations, and practical aspects of regional anesthesia in the trauma patients [7,12–16].

Regional anesthesia techniques for patients who have trauma

Subarachnoid and epidural blockade

Subarachnoid (SAB) and epidural blockade (EB) are by far the regional anesthesia and analgesia techniques most often used in lower limb surgery; recent reports suggest the use of these techniques also to control pain in critically ill patients [6,17–22]. SAB is achieved by the introduction of drugs into the subdural space, whereas EB is achieved by the introduction of drugs into the epidural space. Medications injected epidurally act directly on spinal nerves and receptors in the spinal cord by way of diffusion across the dura and into the cerebrospinal fluid. If minimal sedation is given and a level of anesthesia below the intercostals is maintained, mental status and respiratory function can be well maintained [8].

The more common patient population potentially available for such procedures includes elderly patients who have multiple comorbidities [23] and significant perioperative morbidity and mortality [11,22]. Scheini and colleagues [24] found that a perioperative continuous epidural bupivacaine/fentanyl analgesic regimen reduced the number of myocardial ischemic events in elderly patients who had hip fracture. Recent data suggest that the incidence of severe adverse cardiac events was significantly lower with preoperative epidural analgesia than with standard intramuscular analgesia in patients who had hip fractures [20]. Review of the literature, however, indicates that neither technique offers a significantly better outcome than the other [12], although Urwin and colleagues [13] reported less 1-month mortality in patients receiving regional anesthesia. During replantation and revascularization surgery to date EB does not seem to favor increased blood flow [25].

Cardiovascular instability related to sympathetic block is the most common side effect. Bradycardia and hypotension can be more pronounced with intermittent-bolus dosing in patients who have reduced preload as hypovolemic geriatric patients [8]. These patients often have a pre-existing fluid deficit that is compounded by blood loss from fracture sites into muscular compartments [8]. To avoid hypotension associated with the onset of sympathectomy careful fluid management, with or without the use of invasive monitoring, should be maintained throughout the perioperative period.

A major limitation of epidural analgesia is that it is segmental, needing large volumes of local anesthetics (LAN) to cover extensive injuries (see section dedicated to medications) and the patient's coagulation status.

Recommendations of the American Society of Regional Anesthesia [26] should be followed when considering a patient's coagulation and administration of anticoagulative drugs [27]. Catheter removal must follow the same placement indications. A more extensive review of regional anesthesia and anticoagulation has been published elsewhere [28]. Table 1 [29–31] summarizes indications, contraindications, and practical problems with SAB and EP [6,8,11–13,17–28].

Peripheral nerve blocks

Introduction of new methods and techniques is increasing and improving the use of lower peripheral nerve blocks (PNBs) on the trauma scene. These techniques are also gaining interest after the important increase of the low molecular weight heparins [5,8]. PNBs offer these advantages in the trauma setting: (1) avoid side effects of GA, (2) avoid side effects of neuraxial block, (3) allow rapid and effective analgesia without side effects of systemic analgesics, (4) allow sympathectomy when performed for upper limb surgery with the related advantages in graft surgery [25].

Lower extremities

In patients who have unilateral lower limb fractures who are not candidates for EB regional anesthesia of nerves coming from the lumbar plexus and the sciatic nerve can provide excellent pain relief and good anesthesia at the surgical level. Femoral nerve block or catheters placed with or without the use of an electrical nerve stimulator (ENS) are helpful in the management of acute pain from femoral neck fractures in the perioperative period [32–36] and in prehospital care [37].

Fletcher and colleagues [35] showed that femoral block provides quicker relief than systemic intravenous morphine (5–10 mg/h). The benefit of femoral block was also shown by Lopez and colleagues [37] to facilitate the sitting position for spinal anesthesia.

There are several different techniques that can be used to block the sciatic nerve. Anterior or posterior approach—midgluteal, subgluteal, classic Labat approach—with one or two injections, depends largely on the skills of the operator and the ability to position the patient for the procedure [36–42]. In foot or ankle surgery a popliteal approach might be performed [43].

Table 2 [44] shows indications, contraindications, and practical problems of different types of continuous peripheral nerve blocks in the lower extremities [45–52].

Upper extremities

Upper-limb blocks by way of the brachial plexus are used for laceration repairs, closed reductions, or surgery performed on the arm nerves as a means to prevent neurogenically mediated vasospasm in replantation [25]. Continuous plexus and peripheral nerve blocks offer the potential benefits of prolonged analgesia provided a catheter is positioned [53–62], with fewer side effects, greater patient satisfaction, and faster functional recovery after surgery.

Table 1
Different types of continuous central nerve blocks in the lower extremities

Type of block	Indications	Contraindications	Advised doses	Practical problems and suggestions in trauma patient
Subarachnoid	Orthopedic surgery or trauma of lower extremities	Patient refusal Coagulopathy or current use of anticoagulants, low platelet count [27,28], sepsis/bacteremia [29] Critical aortic stenosis [8] Local infection overlying the needle insertion Severe hypovolemia or acute hemodynamic instability Obstructive ileus Elevated intracranial pressure Pre-existing neuropathy or vertebral trauma Local anesthetic allergies	Surgery: 1.6–2 mL of 0.5 hyperbaric bupivacaine injected over 30 s on L3-L4 and maintaining lateral position for 15 min [30,31] Intrathecal morphine [98,99] injections as single shot or by spinal catheters	Difficult patient positioning, multiple fractures, number and position of tubes and catheters, or external fixation bone devices: another technique should be evaluated Abnormal anatomy: another technique should be evaluated Inability of the patient to cooperate: another technique should be evaluated Hypotension: before the initiation of subarachnoid blockade patients should be carefully hydrated [8]

| Epidural | Orthopedic surgery or trauma of lower extremities | Patient refusal
Coagulopathy or current use of anticoagulants, low platelet count [26–28]
Local infection overlying the needle insertion and sepsis/bacteremia [29]
Severe hypovolemia or acute hemodynamic instability
Obstructive ileus
Elevated intracranial pressure
Pre-existing neuropathy or vertebral trauma
Local anesthetic allergies | Surgery:
10–15 mL of 0.75% ropivacaine ± 10 μg of sufentanil or 10–15 mL of 0.5% bupivacaine ± 10 μg of sufentanil on L4-L5 [98]
Postoperative analgesia:
Bolus regimen:
5–10 mL of 0.125%–0.25% bupivacaine or 0.1%–0.2% ropivacaine every 8–12 h
Consider addition of 1 μg/kg of clonidine in hemodynamically stable patients
Continuous infusion:
0.0625% bupivacaine or 0.1% ropivacaine at 5 mL/h
Consider addition of opioids (eg, hydromorphone, sufentanil) or clonidine if high systemic opioid demands persist | Difficult patient positioning and catheter tunneling: another technique should be evaluated
Abnormal anatomy: another technique should be evaluated
Inability of the patient to cooperate: another technique should be evaluated |

Table 2
Different types of continuous peripheral nerve blocks in the lower extremities

Type of block	Indications	Contraindications	Advised doses[a]	Practical problem and suggestions in trauma patient
Femoral or sciatic nerve	Unilateral leg surgery when both fields of innervation are blocked. Analgesia in their field of innervation when single blocked.	Patient refusal Local infection overlying the needle insertion Pre-existing neuropathy Local anesthetic allergies	Surgery: 10–15 mL of 0.75% ropivacaine or 10–15 mL of 0.5% bupivacaine or 10–15 mL of 2% mepivacaine for femoral nerve block 15 mL of 0.75% ropivacaine or 15 mL of 0.5% bupivacaine or 15 mL of 2% mepivacaine for sciatic nerve block [44] Consider addition of 1 μg/kg of clonidine in hemodynamically stable patients [45,47] Postoperative analgesia: Bolus regimen: 10 mL of 0.25% bupivacaine or 0.2% ropivacaine every 8–12 h and on demand Continuous infusion: 0.125% bupivacaine or 0.1%–0.2% ropivacaine at 5 mL/h [6,59]	Difficult patient positioning: all possible technical approaches should be evaluated Obese patient: all possible technical approaches should be evaluated Interference of femoral nerve catheters with femoral catheters (central venous catheter, arterial catheters) wounds or other alterations of site of puncture: another technique should be evaluated Pain because of ENS: skilled use of ultrasound [50], fascia iliaca compartment block, or small doses of intravenous remifentanil (0.3–0.5 g/kg) or ketamine (0.2–0.4 mg/kg) [11] might limit the unavoidable [6]. Target sedation score Ramsey = 2 [51]
Posterior tibial and popliteal sciatic nerve	Unilateral foot surgery	Patient refusal Local infection overlying the needle insertion Pre-existing neuropathy Local anesthetic allergies	Surgery: 15–20 mL of 0.75% ropivacaine or 15–20 mL of 0.5% bupivacaine or 15–20 mL of 2% mepivacaine [52]	Patient positioning: another technical approach should be evaluated

[a] Maximal dose for single administration: mepivacaine 7 mg/Kg (max 1000 mg/24 h), bupivacaine 2 mg/kg (max 150 mg for single administration), levobupivacaine 150 mg (max 400 mg/24 h), ropivacaine 300 mg (max 675 mg/h).

In upper extremity surgery either interscalene, axillary, or supraclavicular/infraclavicular and cervical paravertebral approaches to the brachial plexus block can be used for anesthesia and also for continuous analgesia [7,53–73]. Interscalene block provides the most reliable anesthesia for shoulder pain and surgery [53–56]. For most authors a continuos block is the analgesia technique of choice, providing better pain control than patient-controlled analgesia with morphine [57,58]. The modified approach by Boezart and colleagues [53] seems to reduce the incidence of catheter dislodgement.

Although it has been demonstrated that patient-controlled analgesia with opioid produces similar effects on pulmonary function as the ipsilateral interscalene block [59], the major limitation of the interscalene block is the unavoidable blocking of the phrenic nerve and the loss of hemidiaphragmatic activity [56].

Infraclavicular and axillary blocks are able to provide good anesthesia levels for surgery of the upper extremities. The continuous infraclavicular and axillary [54,55,64–73] approaches also provide a good level of analgesia during the perioperative period and even days after surgery in patients who need surgical anesthesia for painful wound dressing changes or debridements for major burns [7]. For this reason a catheter positioning instead of single shot technique must be considered. The supraclavicular approach has been almost abandoned because of related high frequency of pneumothorax.

Table 3 [74,75] shows indications, contraindications, and practical problems of different types of continuous peripheral nerve blocks in the upper extremities [76,77].

Analgesia techniques for chest pain

The main advantages to reducing chest pain beyond leaving the patient feeling more comfortable are: (1) to improve respiratory function by decreasing pain on inspiration, allowing deep breath; (2) to allow upright or sitting position [78]; (3) to improve coughing efficacy with decreased risk for atelectasis, hypoxemia, and associated morbidity and mortality [79,80].

Based on current evidence it is difficult to recommend a single method that can be used safely and effectively for analgesia in patients who have multiple fractured ribs [81]. Epidural analgesia has been used after thoracotomy or for multiple rib fractures [80–86] and has been shown to be an independent predictor of decreased morbidity and mortality in thoracic trauma [85] along with improving outcomes in patients who have rib fractures [3].

When EP is contraindicated, intrapleural catheters [86] and thoracic paravertebral catheters [87] can be used as an alternative to epidural catheters for the management of unilateral pain, for rib fractures after chest trauma, or for chest surgery. The major limitations of these techniques is that paravertebral catheters can control pain restricted to a few dermatomes, whereas intrapleural catheters are of limited value secondary to concurrent drainage

Table 3
Different type of continuous peripheral nerve blocks in the upper extremities

Type of block	Indications	Contraindications	Advised doses[a]	Practical problems and suggestions in trauma patient
Interscalene	Shoulder/arm surgery	Patient refusal Untreated contralateral pneumothorax Dependence on diaphragmatic breathing Contralateral vocal cord palsy Local infection overlying the needle insertion Patients who have reduced functional residual capacity, aged patients who have chest trauma or difficult-to-wean patients [7,22] Pre-existing neuropathy Local anesthetic allergies	Surgery: 20–30 mL of 0.5% ropivacaine or 20–30 mL of 0.5% levobupivacaine; 15 mL of 0.5 ropivacaine + GA or 10–15 mL of 0.125% bupivacaine + GA [76] Postoperative analgesia: Bolus regimen: 10 mL of 0.25% bupivacaine or 0.2% ropivacaine every 8–12 h and on demand Continuous infusion: 0.125% bupivacaine or 0.1%–0.2% ropivacaine at 5 mL/h [7]	Block of ipsilateral phrenic nerve: see contraindications Horner syndrome: may obscure neurologic assessment; diagnostic differential diagnosis with head trauma must be carefully evaluated Close proximity to tracheostomy and jugular vein catheter sites [7]: use of the cervical paravertebral approach should be considered [61,62] to reduce the risk for infection Risk for accidental subdural injection [63]: combination of ultrasound and nerve stimulation should be used in sedated patients [66] Risk for accidental arterial/venous/nerve injury

Infraclavicular/ supraclavicular	Forearm/hand surgery	Patient refusal Severe coagulopathy Untreated contralateral pneumothorax Local infection overlying the needle insertion Pre-existing neuropathy Local anesthetic allergies	Surgery: 20–30 mL of 0.5% ropivacaine or 20–30 mL of 0.5% levobupivacaine; 15 mL of 0.5 ropivacaine + GA or 10–15 mL of 0.125% bupivacaine + GA [76] Postoperative analgesia: Bolus regimen: 10–20 mL of 0.25% bupivacaine or 0.2% ropivacaine every 8–12 h and on demand Continuous infusion: 0.125% bupivacaine or 0.1%–0.2% ropivacaine at 5–10 mL/h [7]	Pneumothorax risk: see contraindications Interference with subclavian central venous catheters A lateral infraclavicular approach [60–62] might help to reduce the risk for pneumothorax Risk for accidental arterial/venous injury and risk for arteriovenous fistula: use of ultrasound should be evaluated
Axillary	Forearm/hand surgery	Patient refusal Local infection overlying the needle insertion Pre-existing neuropathy Local anesthetic allergies	Surgery: 20–40 mL of 0.5% ropivacaine or 20–40 mL of 0.5% bupivacaine [73] Postoperative analgesia: Bolus regimen: 10–20 mL of 0.25% bupivacaine or 0.2% ropivacaine every 8–12 h and on demand Continuous infusion: 0.125% bupivacaine or 0.1%–0.2% ropivacaine at 5–10 mL/h [7]	Arm positioning Not suitable for catheter positioning
Cervical paravertebral	Shoulder/arm surgery	Patient refusal Local infection overlying the needle insertion Pre-existing neuropathy Local anesthetic allergies	Surgery: 30 mL of 0.25% bupivacaine Postoperative analgesia: Continuous infusion: 0.25% bupivacaine 5 mL/h [74]	Risk for accidental arterial/venous injury Risk for accidental subarachnoid 1 injection

(continued on next page)

Table 3 (*continued*)

Type of block	Indications	Contraindications	Advised doses[a]	Practical problems and suggestions in trauma patient
Stellate ganglion	Arm/hand vascular surgery	Patient refusal Untreated contralateral pneumothorax Contralateral vocal cord palsy Local infection overlying the needle insertion Local anesthetic allergies	Selective sympathetic nervous system block: 8–10 mL of 1% lidocaine or 0.25% bupivacaine [75]	Risk for accidental vertebral arterial injection Risk for accidental subarachnoid injection Pneumothorax Hoarseness from recurrent laryngeal nerve paralysis
Medianum/radial/ulnar nerve block	Hand surgery	Patient refusal Local infection overlying the needle insertion Pre-existing neuropathy Local anesthetic allergies	Surgery 5–10 mL 0.5% ropivacaine or 5–10 mL of 0.5% bupivacaine [73]	—

[a] Maximal dose for single administration: mepivacaine 7 mg/Kg (max 1000 mg/24 h), bupivacaine 2 mg/kg (max 150 mg for single administration), levobupivacaine 150 mg (max 400 mg/24 h), ropivacaine 300 mg (max 675 mg/h).

from chest tubes [7]. Intercostal nerve block is an effective form of analgesia, and for most patients who have rib fractures one intercostal nerve block is sufficient to allow adequate respiratory exercise and discharge from the hospital [88]. The incidence of pneumothorax per individual intercostal nerve blocked is low.

Other analgesia techniques

Continuous lumbar plexus block may provide relief for acute postoperative pain management after open reduction and internal fixation of acetabular fracture [89]. Celiac plexus blocks may provide excellent analgesia for pancreatitis secondary to trauma but technical difficulties (computed tomography guidance, fluoroscopy, or transgastric ultrasound) and the need for repeated injections limit its use [7]. Single-shot nerve blocks, such as scalp block for the placement of halo fixation, vascular approaches are often forgotten although easy and safe to perform [7,90]. Topical anesthesia can be achieved with Lidocaine-Prilocaine cream (EMLA, AstraZeneca, London). It needs to be applied 30–45 mins before the procedure to achieve an optimal effect [7].

Practical aspects of regional anesthesia in patients who have trauma

Medications

The most frequently used medications for regional analgesia or anesthesia are LAN injected neuraxially or during peripheral nerve blocks, which arrest nerve conduction by way of the blockade of sodium channels. As a consequence, they block the transmission of nerve fibers, not just the A-delta and C fibers responsible for pain. LAN have been shown to have dose-dependent negative effects, such as neurotoxicity, cardiotoxicity, and central nervous excitation or depression, and other side effects not related to dosage quantity, such as myotoxicity and inhibition of wound healing [90,91].

Because of traumatic disease plasma levels on anesthetic can change in critically ill patients [92]. Ropivacaine has been demonstrated to have lower toxicity when compared with bupivacaine and it is indicated for scheduled or long surgery [93–95].

The other most commonly used drugs for epidural analgesia are opioids [96,97]. They act through mu, kappa, and delta receptors in the substantia gelatinosa of the spinal cord. One advantage of epidural opioids over the local anesthetics is the lack of autonomic and motor blockade. In addition, because a major limitation of epidural analgesia is that it is segmental and requires large volumes of LAN, hydrophilic drugs, such as morphine, exhibit greater segmental spread and result in better pain relief than lipid-soluble drugs [98,99]. Because of the 10-fold reduction in equianalgesic doses of opioids between the epidural and intravenous routes, prevalence of certain side effects, such as sedation and constipation, during neuraxial administration is reduced [6]. Unfortunately, greater rostral spread also results in a higher prevalence of side effects [33] and pruritus is more common with the neuraxial route [97]. Complications attributable to high systemic doses of opioids also include sleep disorders, delirium, mental status changes, gastrointestinal dysfunction, and withdrawal syndrome. During PNBs addition of 50 to 150 μg of clonidine in a hemodynamically stable patient or 150 to 300 μg of buprenorphine [45,100] to prolong duration of action may be considered, although there is still controversy in peripheral blocks [46,47]. Clonidine has also been used in neuraxial blocks [48].

A prospective study demonstrated that pain assessment increased the likelihood of analgesic administration to trauma patients [101]. Pain severity scores seem to be underused, however [102]. During the perioperative period preemptive analgesia to reduce the magnitude and duration of postoperative pain shows evidence for a central component of postinjury pain hypersensitivity not only in experimental studies but also in clinical trials [103].

Catheter placement and maintenance

The safety of placing epidural catheters in critically ill patients is related to the level of the patient's consciousness, systemic inflammatory response status, hemodynamic stability, and coagulation, and the use of any anticoagulant medications or antiplatelet drugs [15–17,23,26–28,104]. Regarding the patient's coagulation status, catheter removal must follow the same placement indications [27,28]. Diagnostic approaches, including computed tomography imaging and magnetic resonance, should be considered in the presence of clinical or warning signs of possible bleeding complications.

To prevent local anesthetic side effects from accidental intravascular injection aspiration is strongly suggested during catheter placement to check for blood return and a test dose of local anesthetic or saline with 1:200,000 epinephrine. Because of the traumatic underlying disease and related use of cardiovascular drugs (ie, β blockers, α-2 agonists, catecholamines), cardiovascular parameters, such as heart rate, blood pressure, and ECG changes [94], might be altered. Premedication and deep sedation can also mask side effects [105].

The correct position of the epidural catheter can be achieved by electrical stimulation during placement or a postplacement radiograph with a small amount of non-neurotoxic contrast [106,107].

The routine neurologic daily assessment for long-term catheter can be performed by bolus injections of long-acting local anesthetics, such as bupivacaine, ropivacaine, or levobupivacaine, or the discontinuation of continuous infusions [5,7].

Use of subarachnoid microcatheters, currently not approved in the United States but approved in Europe, can be an alternative to epidural catheters, especially if only short-term use after surgery is anticipated [7].

Catheters suitable for use with ENS should never be cut because of the danger of unwinding the internal metal spiral wire that conducts current. No study has looked at the risk for reconnecting these catheters after thorough disinfection of the outer surface [7]. Regarding incidence of colonization, Cuvillon and colleagues [108] reported a high overall incidence (57%) of femoral catheters without septic complications. The authors concluded that the decision to reconnect or remove the catheter must be based on the individual clinical situation [7]. Catheters should not be removed routinely after a certain span of time but only when clinical signs of infection appear [7,109].

Structured observations of catheters for infectious complications and careful adherence to aseptic technique during placement and tunneling of the catheters, along with the possible use of antibiotic-coated catheters in the future, may reduce possible infectious complications [7].

There is no algorithm for the management of postoperative nerve injury. Most often, symptoms are first noted and referred to as an anesthetic complication by anesthesiologists. Most frequently, residual dysesthesia or hypoesthesia is reported.

Summary

Although no distinct advantage is apparent between regional and general anesthesia, preoperative epidural analgesia or continuous nerve blocks for upper limb amputations and for patients who are poor candidates for neuraxial anesthesia should be strongly considered for injury limited to a limb. This consideration is most important whenever the regional anesthesia techniques are extended into the postoperative period to provide analgesia.

Because of limited patient cooperation, high-quality nursing care and well-trained anesthesiologist are mandatory prerequisites for the use of regional anesthesia safely in all the perioperative period.

References

[1] Cordell WH, Keene KK, Giles BK, et al. The high prevalence of pain in emergency medical care. Am J Emerg Med 2002;20(3):165–9.
[2] Cuthbertson BH, Hull A, Strachan M, et al. Post-traumatic stress disorder after critical illness requiring general intensive care. Intensive Care Med 2004;30:450–5.
[3] Bulger EM, Edwards Thomas, Klotz PRN, et al. Epidural analgesia improves outcome after multiple rib fractures. Surgery 2004;2:426–30.
[4] Osinowo OA, Zahrani M, Softah A. Effect of intercostal nerve block with 0.5% bupivacaine on peak expiratory flow rate and arterial oxygen saturation in rib fractures. J Trauma-Injury Infection & Critical Care 2004;56(2):345–7.
[5] Davidson EM, Ginosar Y, Avidan A. Pain management and regional anaesthesia in the trauma patient. Curr Opin Anaesthesiol 2005;18:169–74.
[6] Cohen SP, Christo PJ, Moroz L. Pain management in trauma patients. Am J Phys Med Rehabil 2004;83:142–61.

[7] Schulz-Stübner S, Boezaart A, Hata JS. Regional analgesia in the critically ill. Crit Care Med 2005;33:1400–7.

[8] Taboada M, Atanassoff PG. Lower extremity nerve blocks. Curr Opin Anaesthesiol 2004; 17:403–8.

[9] Singelyn FJ, Capdevila X. Regional anesthesia for orthopaedic surgery. Curr Opin Anaesthesiol 2001;14:733–40.

[10] Rodgers A, Walker N, Schug S, et al. Reduction of postoperative mortality and morbidity with epidural or spinal anaesthesia: result from overview of randomised trials. Br Med J 2000;321:1493.

[11] O'Hara DA, Duff A, Berlin JA, et al. The effect of anesthetic technique on postoperative outcomes in hip fracture repair. Anesthesiology 2000;92:947–57.

[12] Breen P, Park KW. General anesthesia versus regional anesthesia. Int Anesthesiol Clin 2002;40(1):61–71.

[13] Urwin SC, Parker MJ, Griffiths R. General versus regional anaesthesia for hip fracture surgery: a meta-analysis of randomized trials. Br J Anaesth 2000;84:450–5.

[14] Pasero C, McCaffery M. Multimodal balanced analgesia in the critically ill. Crit Care Nurs Clin North Am 2001;13:195–206.

[15] Auroy Y, Benhamou D, Bargues L, et al. Major complications of regional anesthesia in France: the SOS regional anesthesia hotline service. Anesthesiology 2002;97:1274–80.

[16] Auroy Y, Narchi P, Messiah A, et al. Serious complications related to regional anesthesia: results of a prospective survey in France. Anesthesiology 1997;87:479–86.

[17] Moen V, Dahlgren N, Irestedt L. Severe neurological complications after central neuraxial blockades in Sweden 1990–1999. Anesthesiology 2004;101:950–9.

[18] Wu CL, Anderson GF, Herbert R, et al. Effect of postoperative epidural analgesia on morbidity and mortality after total hip replacement surgery in medicare patients. Reg Anesth Pain Med 2003;28:271–8.

[19] Naber L, Jones G, Halm M. Epidural analgesia for effective pain control. Crit Care Nurse 1994;14:69–72, 77–85.

[20] Matot I, Oppenheim-Eden Arieh, Ratrot R, et al. Preoperative cardiac events in elderly patients with hip fracture randomized to epidural or conventional analgesia. Anesthesiology 2003;98(1):156–63.

[21] De Leon-Casasola OA, Lema MJ, Karabella D, et al. Postoperative myocardial ischemia: epidural versus intravenous patient-controlled analgesia. A pilot project. Reg Anesth 1995; 20:105–12.

[22] Deiner S, Jeffrey H, Silverstein JH, et al. Management of trauma in the geriatric patient. Curr Opin Anaesthesiol 2004;17(2):165–70.

[23] Krane EJ, Dalens BJ, Murat I, et al. The safety of epidurals placed during general anesthesia. Reg Anesth Pain Med 1998;23:433–8.

[24] Scheini H, Virtanen T, Kenatala E, et al. Epidural infusion of bupivacaine and fentanyl reduces perioperative myocardial ischaemia in elderly patients with hip fracture: a randomized controlled trial. Acta Anaesthesiol Scand 2000;44:1061–70.

[25] Taras JS, Behrman MJ. Continuous peripheral nerve block in replantation and revascularization. J Reconstr Micrs 1998;14:17–21.

[26] Kaplan R. ASRA consensus statements for anticoagulated patients. American Society of Regional Anesthesia. Reg Anesth Pain Med 1999;24:477–8.

[27] Horlocker TT, Wedel DJ, Benzon H, et al. Regional anesthesia in the anticoagulated patient: defining the risks (the second ASRA Consensus Conference on Neuraxial Anesthesia and Anticoagulation). Reg Anesth Pain Med 2003;28:172–97.

[28] Krombach JW, Oguzhan D, Kampe S. Regional anesthesia and coagulation. Curr Opinion Anesthesiol 2004;17:427–33.

[29] Wegeforth PLJ. Lumbar puncture as a factor in the pathogenesis of meningitis. Am J Med Sci 1919;158:183–202.

[30] Cappelleri G, Aldegheri G, Danelli G, et al. Spinal anesthesia with hyperbaric levobupivacaine and ropivacaine for outpatient knee arthroscopy: a prospective, randomized, double-blind study. Anesth Analg 2005;101(1):77–82.

[31] Casati A, Fanelli G, Cappelleri G, et al. Effects of spinal needle type on lateral distribution of 0.5% hyperbaric bupivacaine. Anesth Analg 1998;87:355–9.

[32] Finlayson BJ, Underhill TJ. Femoral nerve block for analgesia in fractures of the femoral neck. Arch Emerg Med 1988;5:173–6.

[33] Tan TT, Coleman MM. Femoral blockade for fractured neck of femur in the emergency department. Ann Emerg Med 2003;42:596–7.

[34] Cuignet O, Pirson J, Boughrouph J, et al. The efficacy of continuous fascia iliaca compartment block for pain management in burn patients undergoing skin grafting procedures. Anesth Analg 2004;98:1077–81.

[35] Fletcher AK, Rigby AS, Heyes FL. Three-in-one femoral nerve block as analgesia for fractured neck of femur in the emergency department: a randomized, controlled trial. Ann Emerg Med 2003;41:227–33.

[36] Kaden V, Wolfel H, Kirsch W. [Experiences with a combined sciatic and femoral block in surgery of injuries of the lower leg]. Anaesthesiol Reanim 1989;14:299–303 [in German].

[37] Lopez S, Gros T, Bernard N, et al. Fascia iliaca compartment block for femoral bone fractures in prehospital care. Reg Anesth Pain Med 2003;28:203–7.

[38] Sia S, Pelusio F, Barbagli R, et al. Analgesia before performing a spinal block in the sitting position in patients with femoral shaft fracture: a comparison between femoral nerve block and intravenous fentanyl. Anesth Analg 2004;99:1221–4.

[39] Barbero C, Fuzier R, Samii K. Anterior approach to the sciatic nerve block: adaptation to the patient's height. Anesth Analg 2004;98:1785–8.

[40] Franco CD. Posterior approach to the sciatic nerve in adults: is Euclidean geometry still necessary? Anesthesiology 2003;98:723–8.

[41] Di Benedetto P, Casati A, Bertini L, et al. Posterior subgluteal approach to block the sciatic nerve: description of the technique and initial clinical experiences. Eur J An-aesthesiol 2002; 19:682–6.

[42] Bailey SL, Parkinson SK, Little WL, et al. Sciatic nerve block. A comparison of single versus double injection technique. Reg Anesth 1994;19:9–13.

[43] Connolly C, Coventry D, Wildsmith J. Double-blind comparison of ropivacaine 7.5 mg ml^{-1} with bupivacaine 5 mg ml^{-1} for sciatic nerve block. Br J Anaesth 2001;86:674–7.

[44] Fanelli G, Casati A, Beccaria P, et al. A double-blind comparison of ropivacaine, mepivacaine during sciatic and femoral nerve. Anesth Analg 1998;87:597–600.

[45] Casati A, Magistris L, Fanelli G, et al. Small-dose clonidine prolongs postoperative analgesia after sciatic-femoral nerve block with 0.75% ropivacaine for foot surgery. Anesth Analg 2000;91:388–92.

[46] Murphy D, McCartney C, Chan V. Novel analgesic adjuncts for brachial plexus block: a systematic review. Anesth Analg 2000;90:1122–8.

[47] Mannion S, Hayes I, Loughnane F, et al. Intravenous but not perineural clonidine prolongs postoperative analgesia after psoas compartment block with 0.5% levobupivacaine for hip fracture surgery. Anesth Analg 2005;100:873–8.

[48] De Kock M, Gauthier P, Fanard L, et al. Intrathecal ropivacaine and clonidine for ambulatory knee arthroscopy. A dose–response study. Anesthesiology 2001;94:574–8.

[49] Capdevila X, Pirat P, Bringuier S, et al. Continuous peripheral nerve blocks in hospital wards after orthopedic surgery. Anesthesiology 2005;103:1035–45.

[50] Marhofer P, Schrogendorfer K, Koinig H, et al. Ultrasonographic guidance improves sensory block and onset time of three-in-one blocks. Anesth Analg 1997;85:854–7.

[51] Janzen PR, Hall WJ, Hopkins PM. Setting targets for sedation with a target-controlled program. Anaesthesia 2000;55:666–9.

[52] Casati A, Fanelli G, Koscielniak-Nielsen Z, et al. Using stimulating catheters for continu-
     ous sciatic nerve block shortens onset time of surgical block and minimizes postoperative
     consumption of pain medication after hallux valgus repair as compared with conventional
     nonstimulating catheters. Anesth Analg 2005;101(4):1192–7.
[53] Boezaart AP, de Beer JF, du Toit C, et al. A new technique of continuous interscalene nerve
     block. Can J Anaesth 1999;46:275–81.
[54] Brown DL. Brachial plexus anesthesia: an analysis of options. Yale J Biol Med 1993;66:
     415–31.
[55] Ilfeld BM, Enneking FK. Brachial plexus infraclavicular block success rate and appropriate
     endpoints. Anesth Analg 2002;95:784.
[56] Sala-Blanch X, Lazaro JR, Correa J, et al. Phrenic nerve block caused by interscalene bra-
     chial plexus block: effects of digital pressure and a low volume of local anesthetic. Reg
     Anesth Pain Med 1999;24:231–5.
[57] Borgeat A, Tewes E, Biasca N, et al. Patient-controlled interscalene analgesia with ropiva-
     caine after major shoulder surgery: PCIA vs PCA. Br J Anaesth 1998;81:603–5.
[58] Lehtipalo S, Koskinen LO, Johansson G, et al. Continuous interscalene brachial plexus
     block for postoperative analgesia following shoulder surgery. Acta Anaesthesiol Scand
     1999;43:258–64.
[59] Borgeat A, Perschak H, Bird P, et al. Patient-controlled interscalene analgesia with ropiva-
     caine 0.2% versus patient-controlled intravenous analgesia after major shoulder surgery:
     effects on diaphragmatic and respiratory function. Anesthesiology 2000;92:102–8.
[60] Boezaart AP, De Beer JF, Nell ML. Early experience with continuous cervical paraverte-
     bral block using a stimulating catheter. Reg Anesth Pain Med 2003;28:406–13.
[61] Boezaart AP, Koorn R, Borene S, et al. Continuous brachial plexus block using the poste-
     rior approach. Reg Anesth Pain Med 2003;28:70–1.
[62] Boezaart AP, Koorn R, Rosenquist RW. Paravertebral approach to the brachial plexus: an
     anatomic improvement in technique. Reg Anesth Pain Med 2003;28:241–4.
[63] Benumof JL. Permanent loss of cervical spinal cord function associated with interscalene
     block performed under general anesthesia. Anesthesiology 2000;93:1541–4.
[64] DeLaunay L, Chelly JE. Indications for upper extremity blocks. In: Chelly JE, editor.
     Peripheral nerve blocks: a color atlas. Philadelphia: Lippincott Williams and Wilkins;
     1999. p. 17–27.
[65] Borene SC, Edwards JN, Boezaart AP. At the cords, the pinkie towards: interpreting
     infraclavicular motor responses to neurostimulation. Reg Anesth Pain Med 2004;29:
     125–9.
[66] Sandhu NS, Capan LM. Ultrasound-guided infraclavicular brachial plexus block. Br
     J Anaesth 2002;89:254–9.
[67] Ang ET, Lassale B, Goldfarb G. Continuous axillary brachial plexus block—a clinical and
     anatomical study. Anesth Analg 1984;63:680–4.
[68] Sia S, Lepri A, Campolo MC, et al. Four injection brachial plexus block using peripheral
     nerve stimulator: a comparison between axillary and humeral approaches. Anesth Analg
     2002;95:1075–9.
[69] Retzl G, Kapral S, Greher M, et al. Ultrasonographic findings of the axillary part of the
     brachial plexus. Anesth Analg 2001;92:1271–5.
[70] Kapral S, Jandrasits O, Schabernig C, et al. Lateral infraclavicular plexus block vs. axillary
     block for hand and forearm surgery. Acta Anaesthesiol Scand 1999;43:1047–52.
[71] Greher M, Retzl G, Niel P, et al. Ultrasonographic assessment of topographic anatomy in
     volunteers suggests a modification of the infraclavicular vertical brachial plexus block. Br J
     Anaesth 2002;88:632–6.
[72] Jandard C, Gentili ME, Girar DF, et al. Infraclavicular block with lateral approach and
     nerve stimulation: extent of anesthesia and adverse effects. Reg Anesth Pain Med 2002;
     27:37–42.

[73] Thompson WL, Malchow RJ. Peripheral nerve blocks and anesthesia of the hand. Mil Med 2002;167:478–82.

[74] Borene SC, Rosenquist RW, Koorn R, et al. An indicator for continuous cervical paravertebral block (posterior approach to the interscalenic space). Anesth Analg 2003;97:898–900.

[75] Barash PG, Cullen BF, Stoelting RK. Peripheral nerve blockade. In: Barash PG, Cullen BF, Stoelting RK, editors. Handbook of clinical anesthesia. Philadelphia: Lippincott-Raven Publishers; 1997. p. 369–71.

[76] Casati Andrea; Fanelli Guido; Chelly JE. Interscalene brachial plexus anesthesia and analgesia for open shoulder surgery: what about pharmacokinetics?: in response:. Anesthesia & Analgesia 2003;2:606.

[77] Silverstein W, Saiyed M, Brown A. Interscalene block with a nerve stimulator: a deltoid motor response in a satisfactory endpoint for successful block. Reg Anesth Pain Med 2000;25:356–9.

[78] Rosenberg AD. Reducing post-traumatic morbidity with pain management. Curr Opinion in Anesthesiology 2000;13:181–4.

[79] Ziegler DW, Agarwal NN. The morbidity and mortality of rib fractures. J Trauma 1994;37:975–9.

[80] Holcomb JB, McMullin NR, Kozar RA, et al. Morbidity from rib fractures increases after age 45. J Am Coll Surg 2003;196:549–55.

[81] Karmakar MK, Ho AMH. Acute pain management of patients with multiple fractured ribs. J Trauma 2003;54:615–25.

[82] Simon BJ, Cushman James, Barraco Robert, et al, for the EAST Practice Management Guidelines Work Group. (Pain management guidelines for blunt thoracic trauma. Journal of Trauma-Injury Infection & Critical Care 2005;59(5):1256–67.

[83] Catoire P, Bonnet F. [Locoregional analgesia in thoracic injuries]. Cah Anesthesiol 1994;42:809–14 [in French].

[84] Asantila R, Rosenberg PH, Scheinin B. Comparison of different methods of postoperative analgesia after thoracotomy. Acta Anaesthesiol Scand 1986;30:421–5.

[85] Wisner DH. A stepwise logistic regression analysis of factors affecting morbidity and mortality after thoracic trauma: effect of epidural analgesia. J Trauma 1990;30:799–804 [discussion: 804–5].

[86] Luchette FA, Radafshar SM, Kaiser R, et al. Prospective evaluation of epidural versus intrapleural catheters for analgesia in chest wall trauma. J Trauma 1994;36:865–9.

[87] Karmakar MK, Critchley LA, Ho AM, et al. Continuous thoracic paravertebral infusion of bupivacaine for pain management in patients with multiple fractured ribs. Chest 2003;123:424–31.

[88] Shanti CM, Carlin AM, Tyburski JG. Incidence of pneumothorax from intercostal nerve block for analgesia in rib fractures. J Trauma 2001;51:536–9.

[89] Chelly JE, Casati A, Al-Samsam T, et al. Continuous lumbar plexus block for acute postoperative pain management after open reduction and internal fixation of acetabular fractures. J Orthop Trauma 2003;17(5):362–7.

[90] Pascal J, Simon PG, Allary R, Passot S, et al. Regional blocking techniques for emergency facial tegument surgery. Br J Anaesth 1999;82(Suppl 1):A353.

[91] Zink W, Seif C, Bohl JR, et al. The acute myotoxic effects of bupivacaine and ropivacaine after continuous peripheral nerve blockades. Anesth Analg 2003;97:1173–9.

[92] Zink W, Graf BM. Local anesthetic myotoxicity. Reg Anesth Pain Med 2004;29:333–40.

[93] Scott DA, Emanuelsson BM, Mooney PH, et al. Pharmacokinetics and efficacy of long-term epidural ropivacaine infusion for postoperative analgesia. Anesth Analg 1997;85:1322–30.

[94] Lefrant JY, de La Coussaye JE, Ripart J, et al. The comparative electrophysiologic and hemodynamic effects of ropivacaine and bupivacaine in anesthetized and ventilated pigs. Anesth Analg 2001;93:1598–605.

[95] Horlocker TT, Kufner RP, Bishop AT, Maxson PM, et al. The risk of persistent paresthesia is not increased with repeated axillary block. Anesth Analg 1999;88:382–7.

[96] Gao F, Waters B, Seager J, et al. Comparison of bupivacaine plus buprenorphine with bupivacaine alone by caudal blockade for post-operative pain relief after hip and knee arthroplasty. Eur J Anaesthesiol 1995;12:471–6.

[97] Jorgensen H, Wetterslev J, Moiniche S, et al. Epidural local anaesthetics versus opioid-based analgesic regimens on postoperative gastrointestinal paralysis, PONV and pain after abdominal surgery. Cochrane Database Syst Rev 2000;CD001893.

[98] Borghi B, Agnoletti V, Ricci A, et al. A prospective, randomized evaluation of the effects of epidural needle rotation on the distribution of epidural block. Anesth Analg 2004;98: 1473–8.

[99] Rawal N, Tandon B. Epidural and intrathecal morphine in intensive care units. Intensive Care Med 1985;11:129–33.

[100] Candido KD, Franco CD, Khan MA, et al. Buprenorphine added to the local anesthetic for brachial plexus block to provide postoperative analgesia in outpatients. Reg Anesth Pain Med 2001;26:352–6.

[101] Silka PA, Roth MM, Moreno G, et al. Pain scores improve analgesic administration patterns for trauma patients in the emergency department. Acad Emerg Med 2004;11:264–70.

[102] Brown JC, Klein EJ, Lewis CW, et al. Emergency department analgesia for fracture pain. Ann Emerg Med 2003;42:197–205.

[103] Møiniche S, Kehlet H, Dahl JB. A qualitative and quantitative systematic review of pre-emptive analgesia for postoperative pain relief the role of timing of analgesia. Anesthesiology 2002;96:725–41.

[104] Herwaldt LA, Coffin SA, Schulz-Stübner S. Nosocomial infections associated with anesthesia. In: Mayhall CG, editor. Hospital epidemiology and infection control. 3rd edition. Philadelphia: Lippincott, Williams & Wilkins; 2004. p. 1073–117.

[105] Rosenberg PH, Veering BT, Urmey WF. Maximum recommended doses of local anesthetics: a multifactorial concept. Reg Anesth Pain Med 2004;29:564–75.

[106] Tsui BC, Gupta S, Finucane B. Confirmation of epidural catheter placement using nerve stimulation. Can J Anaesth 1998;45:640–4.

[107] Tsui BC, Guenther C, Emery D, et al. Determining epidural catheter location using nerve stimulation with radiological confirmation. Reg Anesth Pain Med 2000;25:306–9.

[108] Cuvillon P, Ripart J, Lalourcey L, et al. The continuous femoral nerve block catheter for postoperative analgesia: bacterial colonization, infectious rate and adverse effects. Anesth Analg 2001;93:1045–9.

[109] Langevin PB, Gravenstein N, Langevin SO, et al. Epidural catheter reconnection. Safe and unsafe practice. Anesthesiology 1996;85:883–8.

ELSEVIER
SAUNDERS

Anesthesiology Clin
25 (2007) 117–129

ANESTHESIOLOGY
CLINICS

Initial Trauma Management in Advanced Pregnancy

Yuval Meroz, MD[a], Uriel Elchalal, MD[b], Yehuda Ginosar, BSc, MBBS[a],*

[a]Department of Anesthesiology and Critical Care Medicine, Hadassah Hebrew University
Medical Center, POB 12000, Ein Karem, Jerusalem 91120, Israel
[b]Department of Obstetrics and Gynecology, Hadassah Hebrew University Medical Center,
POB 12000, Ein Karem, Jerusalem 91120, Israel

The pregnant trauma patient presents unique challenges to the anesthesiologist. Initial assessment and treatment must take into account the normal physiologic adaptations to pregnancy of the mother and the fetus, the typical patterns of injury seen in pregnancy, and the maternal and fetal response to trauma. Because trauma management typically involves a broad range of physicians, including emergency physicians, surgeons, anesthesiologists, obstetricians, neonatologists, and intensivists, a multidisciplinary approach is required.

Existing knowledge of trauma management in pregnancy is based mostly on animal studies, retrospective clinical reports, and consensus statements, but infrequently is based on solid evidence. In this article, the authors aim to present practical recommendations for initial trauma resuscitation in pregnancy. They focus on the last trimester, specifically beyond 24 weeks, when the physiologic changes become most significant and the fetus is considered viable, and when, occasionally, the treating physician has to reconcile the conflicting demands of both the mother and the fetus. The reader is referred to several excellent articles on the management of the traumatized pregnant patient [1–5] for a more detailed review of the physiologic changes in pregnancy, mechanisms of injury, effects on pregnancy, and management stratagems past initial care, all of which are beyond the scope of this article.

* Corresponding author.
  E-mail address: yginosar@netvision.net.il (Y. Ginosar).

0889-8537/07/$ - see front matter © 2007 Elsevier Inc. All rights reserved.
doi:10.1016/j.atc.2006.11.001
anesthesiology.theclinics.com

Incidence

In the last quarter of the twentieth century, trauma was the leading cause of maternal death during pregnancy in developed countries [6], accounting for 46% of all maternal deaths. All other causes of maternal death are becoming increasingly rare; maternal death due to trauma is the only cause that is becoming more common [7]. The true incidence of trauma during pregnancy is unknown. Data collected from trauma registries show that trauma occurs in 6% to 7% of all pregnancies [8,9]; however, most injuries are minor, so only 0.3% to 0.4% of all pregnant women are admitted to hospital because of trauma [10]. Many pregnant women are the victims of domestic violence, which frequently is underreported, so the real incidence of trauma in pregnancy is probably higher. A national study of family violence from 1985 [11] reported that 15% of pregnant women were assaulted by their partners; other studies have documented an incidence as high as 30% in some populations [12].

Mechanism and cause of injury

According to the Centers for Disease Control, interpersonal violence is emerging as one of the largest causes of maternal death [13]. Nevertheless, most existing literature and trauma registries in the United States identify road traffic accidents as the leading cause of trauma during pregnancy (among patients who receive prehospital care), accounting for about 55% to 70% of all trauma cases, followed by violence (12%–31%) and falls (10%–22%) [8,14–16]. Penetrating trauma occurred in 10% of all victims and in 24% of casualties with an Injury Severity Score (ISS) higher than eight [14].

The pattern of injury in pregnancy frequently differs from that observed in nonpregnant women. Apart from specific pregnancy-related injuries, such as placental abruption and uterine rupture, pregnant women are more likely to suffer serious abdominal injury than their nonpregnant counterparts, but are less likely to suffer serious head or chest injury [14]. Although seatbelts and helmets were used by only 54% to 66% of pregnant trauma victims, compliance with these safety devices was even worse among nonpregnant casualties [14,15]. The mortality, morbidity, and length of stay were similar among pregnant patients, and matched nonpregnant controls [14]. The main cause of traumatic fetal death is road traffic accidents (82%). The leading causes of all fetal deaths are placental abruption (42%) and maternal death (11%) [17].

Maternal physiology and response to trauma

Although pregnancy is a normal physiologic condition, it is characterized by radical changes in the "nonpregnant" physiology and anatomy of most organ systems [18]. By the third trimester, blood volume is increased by 30% to 50%, whereas red blood cell mass is increased by 15% to 20% only, causing "physiologic anemia" with hematocrit values of 32% to 34%. The level of 2,3-diphosphoglycerate is increased, causing a right-shift of the hemoglobin dissociation curve, thus increasing oxygen release to the fetus [1,19]. The cardiac output is increased by 30% to 50% and the systemic vascular resistance decreases by 20%, whereas the central venous pressure (CVP) and pulmonary artery occlusion pressure are not altered. The heart undergoes significant remodeling, with enlargement of all four chambers, thickening of the left ventricular wall, and development of mild tricuspid, pulmonary, and mitral regurgitation. The pregnant patient would be expected to lose a greater volume of blood before the development of objective signs of hypovolemia than her nonpregnant counterpart. Although this may be protective, it may also delay diagnosis of significant life-threatening injury. Furthermore, even after the development of hypovolemic shock, tachycardia and hypotension may be misinterpreted as being the "normal" physiologic changes of pregnancy. However, even during the third trimester, heart rate increases by only 10 to 15 beats per minute and blood pressure decreases by only 5 to 10 mmHg. Therefore, significant tachycardia or hypotension should not be ignored.

The gravid uterus is about 4.5 kg at term. Normally, the uterine vessels are dilated with low resistance, so the uterine blood flow has minimal autoregulation and depends on adequate maternal arterial blood pressure and unobstructed venous return. During hypotension or hypovolemia, uterine blood flow decreases because of the activation of alpha-adrenergic receptors, shifting blood to the systemic circulation. The pressure of the gravid uterus in the supine position may entirely compress the inferior vena cava, causing a 30% decrease in cardiac output and blocking venous return from the uterus. Additionally, in lower limb or pelvic injury, aortocaval compression increases the venous pressure in the lower body and increases the likelihood of venous bleeding from the injured site. Supine hypotension should be corrected by a 15° left tilt or manual left displacement of the uterus in all pregnant trauma patients [19].

The main pulmonary changes are a 20% increase in oxygen consumption, a 40% increase in minute volume, and a 20% to 25% decreased functional residual capacity [1]. These changes result in a significantly lower oxygen reserve, and mandate supplementary oxygen in all traumatized pregnant patients. The $Paco_2$ is reduced significantly to approximately 28 to 30 mmHg [20] because of the increased minute ventilation; an apparently "normal" $Paco_2$ of 40 mmHg is abnormal in advanced pregnancy. Airway anatomy is changed because of weight gain and edema, making airway management more difficult. Although failed intubation rate is 1:2330 in the general population, it is reported as 1:300 in pregnant women [21].

Renal blood flow is increased by about 50%, so the normal upper limits of blood creatinine and urea are much lower, compared with nonpregnant patients. Therefore, "normal" values in a pregnant patient might indicate impaired renal function [4,22].

Uterine and fetal physiology and response to trauma

Fetal well-being depends on adequate uterine blood flow. Lacking autoregulation, the uterus is very sensitive to changes in maternal blood pressure. Maternal hypovolemia or hypotension cause uterine vasoconstriction and decreased uterine blood flow. Maternal hypoxia might cause fetal hypoxia and acidosis. On the other hand, the fetus is protected from hyperoxic damage while in the uterus, even if the mother is ventilated with 100% oxygen. Based on animal studies, maternal hypocapnia ($Paco_2 < 20$ mmHg) and severe hypercapnia ($Paco_2 > 60$ mmHg) cause uterine vasoconstriction. Hypocapnia and maternal alkalosis not only increase uterine artery resistance, but also reduce oxygen delivery to the placenta by left shift of the hemoglobin dissociation curve, thus increasing its affinity to oxygen [23].

Another factor that decreases uterine blood flow is uterine contractions. Uterine contractions shift 300 to 500 ml more blood to the systemic vessels, thus supporting maternal hemodynamics at the expense of uterine blood flow. The fetal response to hypoxia causes redistribution and "centralization" of the blood toward the fetal brain at the expense of uteroplacental blood flow (thus reducing fetal gas exchange) [24]. Severe fetal hypoxia resulted in lactic acidosis and up to a 1000-fold increase in catecholamine concentrations in an animal model [25].

Risk for fetal loss

Maternal or fetal death are the most serious consequences of trauma. The maternal risk can be predicted by the patient's ISS, just as for nonpregnant patients, but predicting fetal risk is more complicated. In a retrospective study by Shah and colleagues [14], involving 114 injured pregnant patients in a level 1 trauma center, they found higher risk of fetal loss when the mothers were in shock (defined by metabolic acidosis) or had high ISS. High risk of fetal loss was found in cases of severe truncal injury (particularly abdominal) and when vaginal bleeding was present. In their study, the presence of abnormal uterine contractions and abnormal fetal heart rate were not predictors of fetal loss or survival.

The association of fetal loss with high ISS (above 15) or severe abdominal, head, chest, or lower extremity injury was also demonstrated by Ikossi and colleagues [15], who retrospectively analyzed the records of 1195 pregnant trauma victims from the National Trauma Data Bank. However, fetal loss has also been noted with minimal maternal injury. Poole and colleagues [16] performed a retrospective study, analyzing the records of 203 pregnant victims of interpersonal violence. The mean ISS was higher in women with fetal death, but five out of eight fetal deaths occurred without apparent maternal injury (ISS = 0). Fetal death with minor maternal injury was also documented in other series [26,27] that included victims of vehicle accidents. Connolly and colleagues [8] found that individual signs, such as vaginal bleeding, uterine contractions, abdominal tenderness, or even abnormal monitoring, were poor individual predictors for preterm delivery or adverse pregnancy outcome. However, when all these symptoms were absent and when fetal monitoring was normal, no adverse fetal outcomes were noted in any patient in their series.

Prehospital management

Pregnancy should be considered as a possible factor in the trauma management of all women of reproductive age. Where feasible, a brief focused obstetric history should be obtained. If the woman is thought to be pregnant, standard trauma guidelines should be followed. However, aortocaval compression is deleterious to both the mother and the fetus, and the patient should be positioned in a 15° left tilt. This positioning can be performed readily, even if spinal injury is suspected, by placing the patient on a rigid board and tilting the whole board, or by performing continuous manual uterine displacement in the supine position. Ideally, pregnant trauma victims should be transported to a trauma center because of the complex management of these injuries, and because the severity of injury may be underestimated. Physical examination may be misleading; a nontender abdomen should not rule out abdominal injury and minor maternal injury cannot rule out serious fetal injury. Because heart rate increases only 10 to 15 beats per minute and blood pressure normally drops by only 5 to 10 mmHg, any marked tachycardia or hypotension should not be related to normal physiologic changes. Maternal oxygen reserve is limited, so high-flow oxygen should be given using a nonrebreathing mask with reservoir, and oxygen saturation should be monitored continuously. If chest tube insertion is required, it should be placed one or two intercostal spaces higher than usual (as much as 4 cm above its normal position), to avoid possible abdominal injury caused the high position of the diaphragm [1]. Ideally, intubation should be performed early in cases of inadequate oxygenation or ventilation, or to protect the airway. However, because of the increased likelihood of difficult intubation in pregnancy, intubation probably should not be attempted at the prehospital stage, unless strictly needed. Various types of supraglottic airway devices, including the Laryngeal Mask Airway, have proved to be useful in rescue airway management of failed intubation in pregnant women [21].

Early hospital care

A working group of the Eastern Association for the Surgery of Trauma (EAST) has recommended guidelines for the diagnosis and management of injury in the pregnant patient [42]. As soon as the patient arrives in the emergency room, an obstetric consultation and fetal monitoring are required, in addition to standard monitoring and resuscitation protocols. Laboratory tests must be compared with the normal values in pregnancy. These should include coagulation tests because pregnant women are at higher risk to develop disseminated intravascular coagulation in response to traumatic placental abruption. Fibrinogen levels are increased twofold during pregnancy, so even "normal" values should raise suspicion. Rhesus-negative patients should receive anti-D antibody to prevent isoimmunization [2,3]. Gynecologic assessment, including vaginal examination, fetal heart rate monitoring, and obstetric ultrasound is essential; in particular, vaginal bleeding is strongly associated with placental abruption and fetal loss [14]. In cases of fetal distress, adequate maternal hemodynamic resuscitation is the mainstay of intrauterine fetal resuscitation. As maternal cardiac output drops, the mother's vital signs are initially preserved at the expense of uterine blood flow. Therefore, fetal distress might be the first sign of maternal hemodynamic deterioration, making fetal monitoring important as a well-being monitor for both the mother and the fetus. Fetal monitoring should be instituted immediately, even if the mother is stable or the fetus is less than 24 weeks gestational age [1]. Left-tilt or manual uterine displacement should be continued.

Timing of intubation

Airway management is the first priority in all trauma patients. Pregnant patients are a special challenge for several reasons: (1) the incidence of difficult intubation is 17 fold higher in advanced pregnancy, compared with nonpregnant patients; (2) aspiration risk is higher; and (3) risk of hypoxia is increased during intubation because of reduced functional residual capacity and increased oxygen consumption. The fetus is sensitive to changes in the maternal acid-base status. Hypoxia and acidosis might cause direct fetal distress, whereas hyperventilation and alkalosis can reduce uterine blood flow by uterine vasoconstriction and left shift of the hemoglobin dissociation curve. Therefore, considering the combination of limited maternal reserve and the exaggerated fetal response to maternal hypoxia, hypercapnia, and acidosis, it seems reasonable to recommend that tracheal intubation be instituted earlier, if possible, and with less stringent criteria than might be the case for a nonpregnant patient. Where possible, intubation should be performed by an experienced team in the emergency room and the goals of ventilation should be to maintain a high Pao_2 and a $Paco_2$ that is normal for advanced pregnancy (28–30 mmHg) [20]. In intubated patients, blood gases should be checked frequently, so early arterial line placement is usually recommended. No guidelines specifically address airway management in pregnant trauma victims, so management of difficult intubation should rely on understanding maternal physiology [21] and existing difficult airway algorithms, such as the American Society of Anesthesiologists' difficult airway algorithm and its modification for trauma [28,29].

Fluids, vasopressors, and tocolytics

The blood volume of pregnant women is up to 50% greater than prepregnant values. Consequently, the pregnant patient needs to lose more blood before clinically evident signs of hypovolemia appear, by which time she typically requires higher volumes for replacement. The need for control of blood loss and adequate fluid/blood replacement is the paramount concern in these patients. Usually, the vascular compliance is high, and there is no impediment to rapid volume replacement. However, the reduced colloid oncotic pressure of pregnancy may increase the risk of pulmonary edema in overtransfusion, particularly in pre-eclampsia. Monitoring volume status may be inaccurate; data obtained from pregnant patients admitted to intensive care units show poor correlation between central venous pressure and left ventricle filling pressure, so some investigators prefer placing a Swan-Ganz catheter if invasive hemodynamic monitoring is required [30,31]. The authors do not advocate direct central fluid volume monitoring in the initial management of trauma in pregnancy, except in the rare occurrence of unstable hemodynamic status or oliguria in a pregnant trauma patient who has either pre-eclampsia or significant cardiac disease.

Generally, vasopressors do not have a role in treating hypovolemic shock, and the pregnant patient is no exception. Normal-for-pregnancy values of pH and $Paco_2$ should be maintained to prevent fetal distress, which can be induced by either acidosis or alkalosis [23]. However, additional mild hypocapnia (if indicated for treatment of raised intracranial pressure in maternal head injuries, for example) is probably safe to the fetus. The therapeutic range of $Paco_2$ during hyperventilation for raised intracranial pressure in pregnancy is not well-defined, but should not be lower than 24 mmHg [4,20]. Use of mannitol in therapeutic doses has been reported to be safe [4] but is controversial, and caution is needed to avoid hyperosmolarity above 320 mOsmol/l, which may cause fetal dehydration.

The controversies about fluid resuscitation with colloids versus crystalloids, hypotensive resuscitation, and hypertonic saline in the general population [32,33] are beyond the scope of this article, but no evidence suggests a different policy in pregnant patients compared with nonpregnant patients [34].

Intravenous magnesium sulfate and the beta-mimetics are potent tocolytic agents that may be considered occasionally if uterine contractions are noted remote from term. However, it is important to appreciate that uterine contractions may be early signs of placental abruption, and ultrasound should be performed as a first-line investigation before instituting tocolysis. Furthermore, these drugs may exacerbate maternal hypotension by inducing maternal vasodilatation, and invasive blood pressure monitoring is recommended if these drugs are required in trauma. Therefore, these drugs are usually inappropriate in trauma management.

Emergency and perimortem cesarean section in trauma

Emergency cesarean section

Cesarean section may be indicated in the initial trauma management of the injured pregnant patient in response to hemodynamic instability, either to control hemorrhage (placental abruption or uterine rupture) or, occasionally, to enable the exposure and control of nonobstetric intra-abdominal bleeding. Fetal distress may be the initial presenting symptom of placental abruption or uterine rupture; ultrasound examination or abdominal CT should be considered to identify free blood or placental abruption. Isolated fetal indications for cesarean section, such as fetal distress in the absence of placental or uterine injury, are only appropriate indications for surgery in the presence of a viable fetus (greater than 26 weeks gestation) and maternal hemodynamic stability. In the hemodynamically unstable patient who has fetal distress without signs of placental abruption, uterine rupture, or intra-abdominal bleeding, appropriate maternal resuscitation, including fluid administration and the control of hemorrhage, is the best approach to improve intrauterine fetal condition.

Morris and colleagues [35] analyzed the records from nine level 1 trauma centers. Of 441 pregnant trauma victims, 32 underwent emergency cesarean section because of either fetal or maternal distress (but not maternal cardiac arrest; see later discussion). Survival rates were 45% for the infants and 72% for the mothers. Their conclusion was that a fetus with an estimated gestational age of 26 weeks that has cardiac activity is salvageable, irrespective of maternal injury [35].

Perimortem cesarean section

In cases of nontraumatic causes of maternal cardiopulmonary arrest unresponsive to initial resuscitation efforts, resuscitation protocols (Advanced Cardiac Life Support/American Heart Association, American College of Obstetrics and Gynecology [36]) recommend performing a perimortem cesarean section, for both maternal and fetal indications. This recommendation requires that a decision to perform surgery be made within 4 minutes of the onset of unresponsive maternal cardiac arrest, and that surgery be performed immediately (even in the emergency room, if necessary). These recommendations follow those of Katz and colleagues [37] in a landmark paper from 1986. In addition to improving the chance for intact fetal salvage, the performance of perimortem cesarean section evacuates the uterus, thus relieving aortocaval compression, potentially improving maternal venous return, and improving the effectiveness of cardiopulmonary resuscitation. Occasional case reports, both before and after Katz's paper, have described cases of maternal and fetal recovery following perimortem cesarean section. The recommendation of Katz and colleagues [37] was aimed initially at all cases of cardiopulmonary arrest, irrespective of the cause. However, in trauma management, the recommendation to perform perimortem cesarean section has not been generally adopted. Mattox and Goetzl [2], referring to trauma management in pregnancy, wrote in 2003 that, "Perimortem cesarean section is an extremely emotional and often futile exercise...." In 2005, Katz and colleagues [38] published a follow-up review of all the reported perimortem sections reported in the medical literature between 1985 and 2004. The investigators found 38 cases, with 34 infants who survived and 4 infants who survived initially. In many of these cases, maternal status improved dramatically after the operation and 13 of the mothers survived. However, these findings were only relevant in nontraumatic causes of maternal arrest. Of the nine reported cases of perimortem cesarean section performed for maternal trauma, only three infants, and none of the mothers, survived. Based on these findings, Katz and colleagues [38] concluded that perimortem cesarean section in trauma does not improve maternal outcome; as regards fetal outcome, it is much less effective than in nontraumatic cardiopulmonary resuscitation. Consequently, the effectiveness of perimortem cesarean delivery for saving both the mother and fetus in trauma is an unresolved issue.

However, one striking advantage of perimortem cesarean section as a recommendation for maternal resuscitation in nontraumatic cardiac arrest is that it provides a unified approach to both maternal and fetal salvage, thus avoiding the conflict between perceived maternal and fetal interests that previously had complicated maternal resuscitation. In trauma resuscitation, however, perimortem cesarean section may not improve maternal outcome, and, as a consequence, it may be difficult sometimes to know at which point, if any, to "abandon" the mother in favor of the fetus. Without easy answers, individualized clinical judgment remains the best strategy.

Diagnostic imaging and radiation exposure in pregnancy

Focused abdominal ultrasonography for trauma (FAST) has an 83% sensitivity for free peritoneal fluid in pregnant trauma victims [39], and is the first-line diagnostic examination in abdominal trauma. If the FAST examination is equivocal, a diagnostic peritoneal lavage may be considered, especially during the first trimester [18].

Exposure to ionizing radiation in pregnancy is always a concern. The accepted cumulative exposure to the fetus is 5 rad [40]. However, even a 1- to 2-rad exposure might increase the chance of childhood leukemia from

3.6:10,000 to 5:10,000 [41]. Chest radiograph causes a minimal fetal exposure (0.00007 rad), but abdominal CT might expose the fetus to 5 rad or more, so its use in early pregnancy is better avoided, unless absolutely necessary. Chest and head CT are much safer, with fetal exposure of 0.1 rad and 0.05 rad, respectively [40]. In cases of unavoidable exposure of the mother to high levels of ionizing radiation in early pregnancy, it may be appropriate to discuss with the patient the possible termination of the pregnancy, once the mother's condition has stabilized.

Summary

The principles enshrined in existing trauma resuscitation protocols for treating nonpregnant trauma victims should also be applied to the pregnant patient.

In addition to these standard protocols, left tilt of the pregnant patient (or the back board) and supplement oxygen are mandatory. The patient should be treated by a multidisciplinary team, preferably in a trauma center. Early intubation is recommended because of the increased incidence of difficult airway and the reduced maternal oxygen reserve, but should be performed where possible by an experienced physician in the emergency room or operating room. The physician should be aware of the different physiologic and laboratory values in normal pregnancy. Maternal volume status can be difficult to evaluate and invasive monitoring might be needed. Fetal monitoring is important to assess both fetal and maternal welfare, because low uterine blood flow might be an early sign of maternal hypovolemia. Imaging examinations, where indicated, should not be delayed because of possible risk of fetal exposure. Even minor maternal trauma, especially if caused by interpersonal violence, might cause fetal loss.

Appendix 1

Practice management guidelines for the diagnosis and management of injury in the pregnant patient: the EAST Practice Management Guidelines Work Group: recommendations.

A. Level 1

1. There are no Level 1 standards.

B. Level 2

1. All pregnant women > 20 weeks' gestation who suffer trauma should have cardiotocographic monitoring for a minimum of 6 hours. Monitoring should be continued and further evaluation should be performed if uterine contractions, a nonreassuring fetal heart rate pattern, vaginal

bleeding, significant uterine tenderness or irritability, serious maternal injury or rupture of the amniotic membranes is present.
2. Kleihauer-Betke analysis should be performed in all pregnant patients > 12 weeks' gestation.

C. Level 3

1. The best initial treatment for the fetus is the provision of optimum resuscitation of the mother and the early assessment of the fetus.
2. All female patients of childbearing age with significant trauma should have a β-HCG performed and be shielded for X-rays whenever possible.
3. Concern about possible effects of high-dose ionizing radiation exposure should not prevent medically indicated maternal diagnostic X-ray procedures from being performed. During pregnancy, other imaging procedures not associated with ionizing radiation should be considered instead of X-rays when possible.
4. Exposure to less than 5 rad has not been associated with an increase in fetal anomalies or pregnancy loss and is herein deemed to be safe at any point during the entirety of gestation.
5. Ultrasonography and MRI are not associated with known adverse fetal effects. However, until more information is available, MRI is not recommended for use in the first trimester.
6. Consultation with a radiologist should be considered for purposes of calculating estimated fetal dose when multiple diagnostic X-rays are performed.
7. Perimortem Cesarean section should be considered in any moribund pregnant woman of ≥ 24 weeks gestation.
8. Delivery in perimortem cesarean sections must occur within 20 minutes of maternal death but should ideally start within 4 minutes of the maternal arrest. Fetal neurological outcome is related to delivery time after maternal death.
9. Consider keeping the pregnant patient tilted left side down 15 degrees to keep the pregnant uterus off the vena cava and prevent supine hypotension syndrome.
10. Obstetric consult should be considered in all cases of injury in pregnant patients.

References

[1] Shah AJ, Kilcline BA. Trauma in pregnancy. Emerg Med Clin North Am 2003;21:615–29.
[2] Mattox KL, Goetzl L. Trauma in pregnancy. Crit Care Med 2005;33:S385–9.
[3] Tsuei BJ. Assessment of the pregnant trauma patient. Injury 2006;37:367–73.
[4] Penning D. Trauma in pregnancy. Can J Anesth 2001;48:R1–4.
[5] Weinberg L, Steele RG, Pugh R, et al. The pregnant trauma patient. Anaesth Intensive Care 2005;33:167–80.
[6] Fildes J, Reed L, Jones N, et al. Trauma: the leading cause of maternal death. J Trauma 1992; 32:643–5.

[7] Sachs BP, Brown DA, Driscoll SG, et al. Maternal mortality in Massachusetts. Trends and prevention. N Engl J Med 1987;316:667–72.

[8] Connolly AM, Katz VL, Bash KL, et al. Trauma and pregnancy. Am J Perinatol 1997;14: 331–6.

[9] Peckham CH, King RA. A study of intercurrent conditions observed during pregnancy. Am J Obstet 1963;87:609–24.

[10] Lavin JP, Polsky SS. Abdominal trauma during pregnancy. Clin Perinatol 1983;10:423–38.

[11] Council on Scientific Affairs, American Medical Association. Violence against women: relevance for medical practitioners. JAMA 1992;267:3184–9.

[12] Guth AA, Pacther HL. Domestic violence and the trauma surgeon. Am J Surg 2000;179: 134–40.

[13] Chang J, Berg CJ, Saltzman LE, et al. Homicide: a leading cause of injury deaths among pregnant and postpartum women in the United States, 1991-1999. Am J Public Health 2005; 95:471–7.

[14] Shah KH, Simons RK, Holbrook T, et al. Trauma in pregnancy: maternal and fetal outcomes. J Trauma 1998;45:83–6.

[15] Ikossi DG, Lazar AA, Moarabito D, et al. Profile of mothers at risk: an analysis of injury and pregnancy loss in 1,195 trauma patients. J Am Coll Surg 2005;200:49–56.

[16] Poole GV, Martin JN Jr, Perry KG Jr, et al. Trauma in pregnancy: the role of interpersonal violence. Am J Obstet Gynecol 1996;174:1873–7.

[17] Weiss HB, Songer TJ, Fabio A. Fetal deaths related to maternal injury. JAMA 2001;286: 1863–8.

[18] Cunningham FG, Leveno KJ, bloom SL, et al. Maternal physiology. In: Cox SM, Werner CL, Hoffman B, et al, editors. Williams obstetrics. 22nd edition. New York: McGraw-Hill; 2005. p. 121–50.

[19] Fujitani S, Baldisseri MR. Hemodynamic assessment in a pregnant and peripartum patient. Crit Care Med 2005;33(Suppl):S354–61.

[20] Cook PT. The influence on foetal outcome of maternal carbon dioxide tension at caesarean section under general anaesthesia. Anaesth Intensive Care 1984;12:296–302.

[21] Munnur U, Suresh MS. Airway problems in pregnancy. Crit Care Clin 2004;20:617–42.

[22] Yeomans ER, Gilstrap LC III. Physiologic changes in pregnancy and their impact on critical care. Crit Care Med 2005;33(Suppl 10):S256–8.

[23] Shay DC, Bhavani-Shankar K, Datta S. Laparoscopic surgery during pregnancy. Anesthesiol Clin North America 2001;10:57–67.

[24] Li H, Gudmundsson S, Olofsson P. Acute centralization of blood in compromised human fetuses evoked by uterine contractions. Early Hum Dev 2006;82(11):747–52.

[25] Paulick R, Kastendieck E, Weth B, et al. Metabolic, cardiovascular and sympathoadrenal reactions of the fetus to progressive hypoxia-animal experiment studies. Z Geburtshilfe Perinatol 1987;191:130–9.

[26] Agran PF, Dunkle DE, Winn DG, et al. Fetal death in motor vehicle accidents. Ann Emerg Med 1987;16:1355–8.

[27] Esposito TJ, Gens DR, Smith LG, et al. Trauma during pregnancy. A review of 79 cases. Arch Surg 1991;126:1073–8.

[28] American Society of Anesthesiologists Task Force. Practice guidelines for management of the difficult airway. Anesthesiology 2003;98:1269–77.

[29] Wilson WC. Trauma: airway management. Available at: http://www.asahq.org/Newsletters/ 2005/11–05/wilson11_05.html. Accessed November 2005.

[30] Wallenburg HC. Invasive hemodynamic monitoring in pregnancy. Eur J Obstet Gynecol Reprod Biol 1991;42(Suppl):S45–51.

[31] Bolte AC, Dekker GA, van Eyke J, et al. Lack of agreement between central venous pressure and pulmonary capillary pressure in preeclampsia. Hypertens Pregnancy 2000;19:261–71.

[32] Nolan J. Fluid resuscitation for the trauma patient. Resuscitation 2001;48:57–69.

[33] Krausz MM. Initial resuscitation of hemorrhagic shock. World J Emerg Surg 2006;1:14.

[34] Martel MJ, MacKinnon KJ, Arsenault MY, et al. Hemorrhagic shock. J Obstet Gynaecol Can 2002;24:504–20.
[35] Morris JA, Rosenbower TJ, Jurkovich GJ, et al. Infant survival after cesarean section for trauma. Ann Surg 1996;223:481–91.
[36] American College of Obstetricians and Gynecologists (ACOG) educational bulletin. Obstetric aspects of trauma management. Number 251, September 1998. Int J Gynaecol Obstet 1999; 64(1):87–94.
[37] Katz VL, Dotters DJ, Droegemueller W. Perimortem cesarean delivery. Obstet Gynecol 1986;68:571–6.
[38] Katz V, Balderston K, DeFreest M. Perimortem cesarean delivery: were our assumptions correct? Am J Obstet Gynecol 2005;192:1916–21.
[39] Goodwin H, Holmes JF, Wisner DH. Abdominal ultrasound examination in pregnant trauma patients. J Trauma 2001;50:689–93.
[40] Toppenberg KS, Hill DA, Miller DP. Safety of radiographic imaging during pregnancy. Am Fam Physician 1999;59:1813–8.
[41] Brent RL. The effect of embryonic and fetal exposure to x-ray, microwaves, and ultrasound: counseling the pregnant and nonpregnant patient about these risks. Semin Oncol 1989;16: 347–68.
[42] Practice management guidelines for the diagnosis and management of injury in the pregnant patient: the EAST Practice Management Guidelines Work Group. Available at: http://www.east.org/tpg/pregnancy.pdf#search=%22acog%20trauma%20guidelines%22. Accessed June 2005.

ELSEVIER
SAUNDERS

Anesthesiology Clin
25 (2007) 131–145

ANESTHESIOLOGY
CLINICS

Battlefield Anesthesia: Advances in Patient Care and Pain Management

Bruce C. Baker, CAPT, MC, USN[a],[*],
Chester (Trip) Buckenmaier, LTC, MC, USA[b],
Nalan Narine, CDR, MC, USN[a],
Michael E. Compeggie, LCDR, MC, USN[c],
George J. Brand, LT, NC, USN[d],
Paul D. Mongan, COL, MC, USA[e]

[a]Naval Hospital, Camp Pendleton, CA 92055, USA
[b]Walter Reed Army Medical Center, Washington, DC 20307, USA
[c]Naval Hospital, Camp LeJeune, NC 28547, USA
[d]1st Medical Battalion, Camp Pendleton, CA 92054, USA
[e]Department of Anesthesiology, The Uniformed Services University,
Walter Reed Army Medical Center, Washington, DC 20307, USA

Battlefield anesthesia

Battlefield surgery in Iraq has moved ahead light-years compared with previous conflicts (Fig. 1). Despite the increasing lethality of insurgent attacks, the survival percentages of our troops have never been higher. A great part of this is because of improved protective gear—our troops drive armored high-mobility multipurpose wheeled vehicles (Humvees) and other vehicles and wear flak and Kevlar individual armor, ballistic glasses to protect their eyes, and even ballistic ear plugs that reduce the risk for damage to their ears [1–3]. A higher percentage of injuries is to extremities, and more of our troops are surviving to reach the medical surgical help they need to continue to survive [4–6]. Military medicine is traditionally sorted into five levels of care delivery for combat injuries.

The views expressed in this article are those of the authors and do not necessarily reflect the official policy or position of the Department of the Navy, Department of Defense, or the US Government.

The authors have no commercial ties to any of the products mentioned in this article.

* Corresponding author. 5058 Corte Alacante, Oceanside, CA 92057.

E-mail address: bcbaker@cpen.med.navy.mil (B.C. Baker).

1932-2275/07/$ - see front matter. Published by Elsevier Inc.
doi:10.1016/j.anclin.2006.12.003

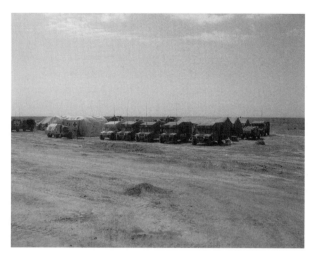

Fig. 1. Forward resuscitative surgical systems and shock trauma platoons deployed in Iraq. (*Courtesy of* Bruce Baker, Oceanside, CA.)

Level 1

Level 1 is up to the level of the battalion aid station, from self-aid and buddy aid to aid by a hospital corpsman or medic (IV, morphine, antibiotics) to mobile emergency room setup, such as the shock trauma platoon (STP). Care at this level is provided by general medical officers or by specialists, depending on the setup, and is mostly advanced trauma life support with some exceptions. Diagnostic equipment can range from virtually nothing except a Propaq, to laboratory and radiograph support, ultrasound, and so forth. Care is modified in the face of tactical or battlefield circumstances and it is now performed with a focus on stopping or limiting hemorrhage (tourniquets and dressings) and hypotensive resuscitative technique [7–12]. Anecdotally, one-handed tourniquets and hemostatic dressings are credited with saving multiple lives. Additional review of treatments and outcomes is required for more definitive conclusions. Fluid resuscitation is given only up to the point of maintaining a blood pressure in the 80 to 90s range, with transport to a location with early surgical intervention being of paramount importance. Airway management at these forward units is currently provided by direct laryngoscopy and endotracheal tube placement or surgical airway as the only two options, and is variable with regard to provider competency. Before deployment, many of the providers brush up on intubating skills in the local military hospitals. The King LT-D is one prehospital modality that some providers are carrying.

Although the initial efforts focus on survival of the soldier, effective pain management is an important consideration because we have realized that pain is more than an unfortunate consequence of wounding and may be a disease process in and of itself [13]. Effective pain control may have positive effects on recovery following trauma and may reduce morbidity over the long term [14]. For more then 200 years, morphine has been the mainstay of battlefield pain management. In the current Iraq conflict the United States military has evaluated the use of fentanyl lollipops with initial success in the treatment of combat casualties [15].

Level 2

The military defines Level 2 as the first level at which surgical intervention is performed. In the Navy this care can be provided by either a surgical company or a forward resuscitative surgical system (FRSS) [16,17]. In the Army the equivalent units are called forward surgical teams and in the Air Force they are known as mobile forward air surgical teams [6].

One or two FRSS teams are usually paired with an STP to form a surgical/shock trauma platoon (SSTP). The STP is staffed by two emergency medicine physicians, physician assistants, nurses, and hospital corpsmen and functions as an emergency department. The addition of the STP gives the unit limited holding capacity. The FRSS teams are made up of either two general surgeons or one general and one orthopedic surgeon, one anesthesia provider, a critical care nurse, a physician assistant, and surgical technicians.

These teams provide surgical care near the forward edge of the battle area. They were designed for expeditionary warfare and the teams can be deployed and ready to receive casualties within an hour. Such care is known as tactical surgical intervention, because it is modified by the physiologic status of the patients and the tactical situations occurring in the battlefield. Other factors that influence clinical decisions include numbers of patients, types of wounds, limited supplies, and medical evacuation time and availability [6,16–18]. Life-and-limb salvage or "damage control" surgery is the norm at these sites. Such surgeries would include revascularization techniques using primary repair or shunts, laparotomies to stop hemorrhage from liver or splenic damage and contamination from bowel injuries, thoracotomies for lung or vascular repair, and extremity wound explorations and possible external fixations of fractures. This type of surgery allows for the stabilization of those patients who would not otherwise survive transport to more distant surgical sites (Fig. 2).

Anesthetic equipment is lightweight, mobile, and able to withstand field conditions. Most surgical cases at this level are performed under general anesthesia. Total intravenous anesthesia (TIVA) can be achieved by way of a Bard infusion pump using ketamine or propofol, but no target controlled infusion capability is currently available. General anesthetics using inhaled agents are still the norm.

Surgical companies are outfitted with the Drager Narkomed M field anesthesia machine. This is a standard anesthesia machine, with a variable

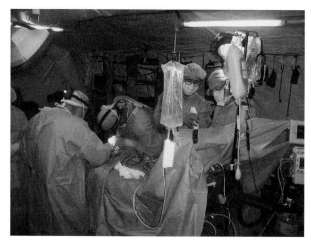

Fig. 2. Forward surgery operating suite. (*Courtesy of* Bruce Baker, Oceanside, CA.)

bypass vaporizer and a gas-driven ventilator. It uses a Venturi-based design to decrease oxygen consumption [19]. It is capable of volume-controlled ventilation. Ventilator drive gas is user selectable to be either oxygen or air.

Modular, lightweight, and rugged, The Narkomed M is well suited for field operations. The major limitation of this machine is high oxygen consumption. With mechanical ventilations and fresh gas flows of 1 L/min gas consumption, the Narkomed M can optimally be driven by approximately 6 L/m oxygen [19]. Practically speaking, when paired with a 10 L/min portable oxygen generator system (POGS), compressed air from the POGS should be used to drive the bellows so that the oxygen reservoir is not depleted. Using compressed gas to drive the bellows and 1 to 2 L/min oxygen for fresh gas flows, even patients who have poor lung compliance or hypermetabolic states can be ventilated.

FRSS and other forward surgical teams are equipped with the Ohmeda Universal Portable Anesthesia Complete (UPAC), more commonly known as the drawover vaporizer. This type of vaporizer was used in the 1973 Yom Kippur war and the 1982 Falkands conflict, and in Somalia, Desert Storm, Afghanistan, and Operation Iraqi Freedom (OIF). The drawover is a variable-bypass, calibrated, temperature-compensated, flow-over, low-resistance, agent-nonspecific vaporizer [20]. The UPAC also compensates for changes in barometric pressure. Compact, lightweight, and rugged, the UPAC meets the needs of these mobile surgical teams. The vaporizer can be used with no supplemental oxygen source applied, and delivers a fraction of inspired oxygen (F_{IO_2}) of 21% [21] consistently. Only with extremely high percentages of end tidal agent (eg, 5% isoflurane) and no supplemental oxygen does the F_{IO_2} fall below 21%. When it is used with supplemental oxygen at 1 to 2 L/min it is capable of delivering F_{IO_2} concentrations of 40% to 50% with the use of oxygen reservoir tubing [22,23]. Isoflurane is the only volatile agent currently used in Level 2 sites, but this vaporizer is also calibrated for use with halothane, enflurane, and diethyl ether. This flexibility is useful when deploying forces may have to depend on host nation supplies of anesthetic agents. Because the vapor pressure of sevoflurane is similar to enflurane it can be used with the drawover. The drawover is capable of delivering only 3% to 4% sevoflurane, however, and so is not optimal for inhalational inductions [24].

The Impact 754 Univent ventilator, which is used at Level 2 facilities, is a lightweight transport ventilator capable of functioning with room air, a high-pressure oxygen source, or low-flow supplemental oxygen. It can operate 3 to 4 hours on its battery and can withstand temperatures of up to 120°F. Exposure to extreme heat can decrease battery life. These ventilators are used for the ICU, patient transport, and in the operating room (OR) with the Ohmeda drawover vaporizer to provide positive pressure ventilation during surgery. The "pull through" method, described in the Emergency War Surgery Manual, is used (Fig. 3) [25]. The ventilator is

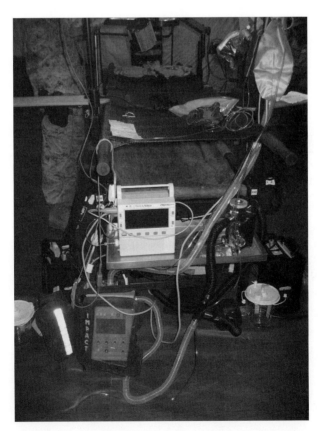

Fig. 3. Impact 754 ventilator with Ohmeda portable anesthesia complete drawover vaporizer. (*Courtesy of* Bruce Baker, Oceanside, CA.)

positioned between the patient and the vaporizer. This position avoids the potential for delivery of anesthetic concentrations greater than the setting on the vaporizer dial when the vaporizer is positioned between the patient and the ventilator [26]. The Univent works well in the OR, is used by all armed services, and is approved for in-flight use. The Univent can function in synchronized intermittent mandatory ventilation, assist-control, or continuous positive airway pressure mode. Tidal volumes, rate, I:E ratio, Fio_2, and pressure limits can be set. Disconnect, low tidal volume, and high or low peak airway pressure alarms are present. One problem when using the ventilator with the vaporizer is that the drawover is calibrated for spontaneous or assisted ventilations, but when combined with the Impact these calibrations are not accurate so the agent delivered can be 0.5% to 1% lower than expected [25,26]. For this reason, an end tidal agent analyzer, such as the VAMOS (Drager Medical) or Cardiocap 5 (Datex-Ohmeda), is recommended (Fig. 4).

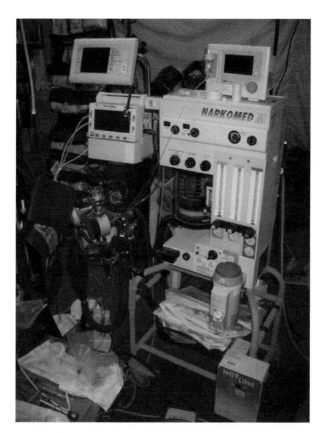

Fig. 4. Narkomed M field anesthesia machine with VAMOS Agent Analyzer. (*Courtesy of* Bruce Baker, Oceanside, CA.)

There are limited blood products available at the Level 2 facilities. Type O+ and O− packed red blood cells (PRBCs) are readily available. Most resuscitations involve some combination of colloid, crystalloid, and PRBCs. Frequently combat trauma patients require massive blood transfusion, and this invariably leads to a dilutional and consumptive coagulopathy. These cases require fresh whole blood using the "walking blood bank." Blood donations are taken from a pool of military members, optimally selected and typed before deployment (because dog tags worn by the Marines have up to a 25% rate of having the wrong blood type), who have the same ABO type-specific blood as the casualty. Most sites in Iraq can also type and cross-match the blood in the laboratory. The blood provides valuable clotting factors, platelets, and red blood cells and is usually considered after about 4 to 6 units of PRBCs. By limiting donors to active-duty military members who receive hepatitis B vaccination with verified titers, HIV screening, and urine drug screening, infectious risks should be minimal. Off-label use of recombinant Factor VIIA (Novo Seven) anecdotally aided in the surgeries of several trauma patients and the authors have heard of no reports of significant complications. The surgical company's laboratory capability can provide type-specific, cross-matched whole blood to the OR within minutes [27].

"Difficult airway" equipment is also limited at Level 2 sites. Initially, the laryngeal mask airway (LMA) was the only nonsurgical rescue option available after failed intubation. Level 2 units were also provided with percutaneous cricothyrotomy kits. Currently lighted stylets, Eschmann intubating stylets, Combitubes, and Intubating LMAs are being used. Fiberoptic bronchoscopes will be available in the future as part of the regular stocked items. Airway trauma has traditionally been noted to be about 1% of total injuries. Facial trauma attributable to penetrating trauma typically is treated with a surgical airway if the patient is in acute distress but in most cases can be intubated by way of direct laryngoscopy. During OIF, the author treated several patients who had anterior airway injuries wherein the laryngeal apparatus was not disrupted and the patients were intubated in a straightforward manner. One patient who had penetrating trauma to the anterior thyroid cartilage presented with dysphonia. The patient was intubated awake with ketamine and midazolam sedation, maintaining spontaneous ventilation with a 6.0 endotracheal tube because of subglottic stenosis of his airway.

Regional anesthesia (neuraxial and peripheral nerve block) along with local anesthesia became an important modality for care in patients who had extremity injuries. At Level 2 facilities the availability of spinal kits, b-bevel insulated needles, and peripheral nerve stimulators could be sought through the logistic supply chain. Approximately 25% of all surgical cases at one Level 2 facility involved regional anesthesia. Most sites have peripheral nerve block capability but no continuous block catheters are available until Level 3. Many patients injured by improvised explosive devices may be injured in multiple extremities, so general anesthetics are performed for most cases (Fig. 5).

With the current static battlefield environment of OIF, the use of regional anesthesia can be beneficial in providing preoperative analgesia or intraoperative anesthesia as a sole anesthetic or combined with general anesthesia. Regional anesthesia provides excellent postoperative analgesia, decreasing the narcotic use and possibly decreasing the incidence of chronic pain syndromes.

Malignant hyperthermia is a relatively rare condition (1:50,000 adult anesthetics reported in North American population) and these patients have extensive intensive care requirements. Because of this, dantrolene was not initially available at Level 2 sites in expeditionary mode and patients experiencing an episode of malignant hyperthermia were to be treated as expectant. Now every Navy Level 2 facility has access to dantrolene.

POGS are used to supply oxygen at Level 2 facilities. The POGS 33/POGS 10 (Onsite Gas) can deliver 33 and 10 L of oxygen (93%–96%) per minute, respectively. Their performance is limited by altitude. The POGS 10 units can run continuously at 10 L/min oxygen production for taking care of patients or refilling oxygen tanks. Oxygen tanks are refilled using the Rix oxygen booster system to compress them up to 2200 psi. An E cylinder takes approximately 75 minutes to refill in this manner using the POGS 10.

Invasive pressure monitoring and noninvasive blood pressure, oxygen saturation, EKG, and end tidal carbon dioxide monitoring are available, and end tidal agent monitoring is being added. Although somewhat limited in the supplies and diagnostic equipment available, such units can do basic laboratories, including complete blood count and arterial blood gases, basic radiographs, abdominal ultrasound exams, invasive monitoring, and mechanical ventilation of patients [28]. In a stationary battlefield, such as Iraq, there are several small surgical units like this spread over the country, with several larger Level 3 hospitals in more central areas.

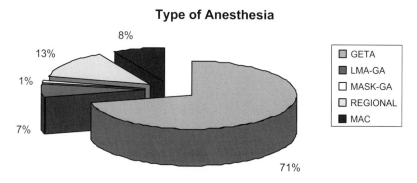

Type of Anesthesia

8%
13%
1%
7%
71%

GETA
LMA-GA
MASK-GA
REGIONAL
MAC

Fig. 5. Types of anesthesia. (*Courtesy of* Bruce Baker, Oceanside, CA.)

In one small study comparing the efficacy of such surgical units with a Level 1 trauma center, such as Los Angeles County, patients who had similar injury severity scores (ISS) sorted into moderate (ISS 16–24) or severe (ISS 25+) were evaluated for outcome and were found to have equivalent chances of survival [29].

En route care

Medical evacuation is usually by helicopter and may be accompanied by en route care (ERC) nurses for the severely injured. Roughly 20% of patients who receive life- saving care at Level 2 facilities are still stabilizing with such life-threatening problems as hypothermia, hypotension, coagulopathy, and airway needs [16]. These patients are still receiving blood products, are intubated and ventilated, and may have vascular shunts and multiple thoracostomy tubes and drains to care for. They are transported by stretcher under the care of specially trained nurses who must care for their patients working out of a single backpack of fluids, medicines, and equipment, often in dark and hazardous conditions. All of the previous efforts of life-and-limb salvage amount to nothing without the expertise and dedication of these flight-trained medical personnel.

The en-route care system (ERCS) is still relatively new and born from necessity during OIF I. The first nurses were picked from various people in the 1st Medical Battalion and nurses at a fleet hospital. During OIF II (year 2 in Iraq), ERC nurses were actually assigned to each medical unit. No real training existed and not all nurses were critical-care trained, however. Finally, the first training pipeline was designed before OIF III (year 3 in Iraq), in which the Navy Operational Medical Institute and the United States Army School of Aviation Medicine started courses.

The ERCS equipment is a continual work in progress, becoming lighter and more compact, to better fit in the various aircraft models available for transport (ie, UH-60, CH-46, CH-53, MV-22, and so forth) The team itself is changing also. Originally designed to be just one nurse, a corpsman is now part of the two-person team (Fig. 6).

The ERCS is slowly coming to maturity. Nurses fly almost daily in Iraq. They use creativity and initiative to come up with new ways to make their kits more useful. Nurses have done everything from adapting equipment from the Army to using specially marked body bags to keep their patients warm. Although currently a Marine Corps program, the Navy and Army are taking a serious look at the ECRS.

Level 3

Level 3 surgical hospitals are designed to be mobile also but take much more time and energy to move. They have six or more ORs and have many

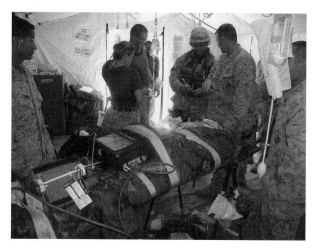

Fig. 6. En route care team preparing to transport a patient. (*Courtesy of* Bruce Baker, Ocean-side, CA.)

different surgical specialties represented, including general, orthopedics, neu-rosurgery, otolaryngology, maxillofacial, ophthalmology, and other special-ists [1,3,30]. The Narkomed M anesthesia machine is used in each OR. Much more advanced therapeutic and diagnostic equipment is available. In an expeditionary battlefield, but also in the stationary operations in Iraq, pa-tients may transfer through each level (1, 2, and 3) before leaving the country. With central coordination of casualty evacuation, however, flights may take a patient to Level 2 facilities for life-and-limb–sparing operations or straight to Level 3 facilities for more specialized (ie, neurosurgical, facial, ophthalmo-logic) care. In prior conflicts, wounded soldiers spent many days to weeks re-covering from wounds in field hospitals before they were considered stable enough for transport back to major hospitals outside of the operational the-ater. Now most patients whose injuries do not allow them to return to duty in 7 days are leaving Iraq from the Level 3 centers within 24 to 48 hours.

Advances in pain management

For more then 200 years, morphine was the mainstay of battlefield pain management. The significant role and advantages of morphine in treating pain in previous conflicts is undeniable. Morphine was an effective tool in previous wars because patients were static in the field hospital and their pain could be managed with scheduled doses of morphine provided by hos-pital nurses. In the present conflict, evacuation of the wounded from Iraq has accelerated with wounded soldiers arriving in a major military hospital (Landstuhl Regional Medical Center, Germany) as soon as 36 to 48 hours after injury. The new goal of field medicine for wounded soldiers is stabilization of the patient for transport to the next level of care. The difficulties in managing pain in this environment are numerous. Multiple providers, communication difficulties over long distances, and austere patient-monitoring conditions are just a few of the issues that limit the usefulness of traditional, morphine-based pain management protocols. The need for new pain management technologies and strategies was recognized early in the Afghanistan and Iraq conflicts. In addition to surgical procedures, many of the patients leaving these centers have either continuous peripheral nerve block infusion catheters placed or patient-controlled analgesia (PCA) devices with them to make the flight out of Iraq more comfortable [31,32]. This is a relatively new addition to the standards of care that can be given to patients recovering from their wartime wounds, and can improve overall patient care tremendously. Because cooperation between the military medical services was necessary to establish a rapid evacuation system for severely injured patients, multiservice pain management of casualties has required extensive coordination. This problem was illustrated by initial difficulties encountered in using continuous blocks in the evacuation system. The infusion pump selected to transport patients (Stryker PainPumpII, Kalamazoo, MI) (Fig. 7), although acceptable in the Army combat support hospitals, was initially not acceptable for use in flight on Air Force military aircraft

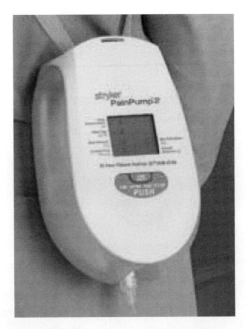

Fig. 7. Stryker PainPumpII currently approved for flight on United States military aircraft for use with continuous peripheral nerve block catheters. (*Courtesy of* Chester Buckenmaier, Gambrills, MD.)

because it had not been tested for compatibility with critical flight systems. This early setback established the need for better tri-service communication if advances in pain management were going to be applied successfully for all three services. Subsequently, the Military Advanced Regional Anesthesia and Analgesia (MARAA) organization was established in 2005. The organization works to develop consensus recommendations from the Air Force, Army, and Navy anesthesia services for improvements in anesthesia practice and technology to promote regional anesthesia and analgesia. Through the efforts of MARAA, the infusion pump was approved for flight and a training program was established to train medical personnel throughout the evacuation system in the use of continuous peripheral nerve block technology in soldiers. Today, continuous nerve bocks are a viable alternative for the anesthetic and analgesic management of combat wounded.

Because the percentage of wounded that were receiving blocks was small, owing to training and wounds that were inappropriate, the use of PCA was more likely to benefit wounded soldiers in combat support hospitals or military flights. Providing PCA technology to patients would reduce pain medication response times and also unburden medical personnel from having to manually provide IV morphine injections, conceivably freeing them to attend more severely injured patients on the flight. After a review of available infusion pump technology, the Sorenson, AmbiT PCA infusion pump was accepted as a temporary solution for PCA. These devices are being used in wounded soldiers throughout their evacuation today (Fig. 8).

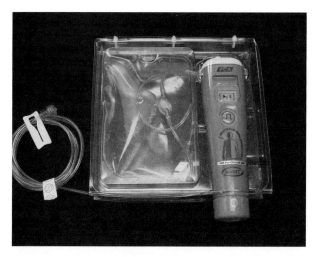

Fig. 8. Sorenson, AmbiT PCA pump currently approved for flight on United States military aircraft for use in morphine PCA. (*Courtesy of* Chester Buckenmaier, Gambrills, MD.)

Level 4

After receiving initial surgeries and pain management in military hospitals in Iraq, patients are transported by Air Force medical evacuation planes to a Level 4 hospital out of the continental United States, such as Landstuhl, Germany. The in-flight capabilities of these transports is akin to a mobile ICU, with trained nursing and intensivist care for the multiple patients requiring specialized intensive care. These medical specialists typically have had Critical Care Aeromedical Evacuation Team training and are well versed in taking care of the critically injured patients coming from Iraq. Some patients who are injured in Iraq awaken for the first time in Landstuhl or even back in the United States, remaining intubated and ventilated through multiple surgeries before regaining full consciousness. The patients are further evaluated and depending on urgency, flight availability, and so forth, may have further surgery there or may be sent on to the United States. Usually the continuous block or PCA techniques are continued throughout this stage and back to the stateside hospitals.

Level 5

Currently patients are flown into the Bethesda/Walter Reed Hospital Consortium near Washington, DC, two of several Level 5 hospitals within the continental United States where further evaluation and treatment are rendered. In some cases, the patients are reaching Bethesda as soon as 48 hours after wounding, although the average is 6 to 7 days [30]. Depending on the injuries immediate care is provided or ongoing restorative care is performed over weeks at these tertiary care centers. Soldiers who have stable wounds that do not need acute or subspecialty care are evaluated and released to return to their local hospitals. The completion of their initial care and such follow-up as needed may occur at these smaller centers or through the Veteran's Affairs system, depending on the patient's duty status and disability. Routine screening for posttraumatic stress disorder and chronic pain is occurring at each of these sites.

Summary

Expeditionary maneuver warfare and the asymmetric battlefield have forced changes in the traditional methods with which we deliver anesthesia and surgery to the wounded. Although in many ways similar to how we have operated on the wounded for the past half century, new advances in diagnostic and therapeutic modalities and doctrinal shifts have changed the face of the battlefield hospital. Advances in pain management have increased the ability to care for injured patients, while movement of casualties from the battlefield back to facilities in the United States has accelerated tremendously, allowing for specialized care much sooner then previously. These advances should result in improvements in morbidity and mortality for wounded veterans.

References

[1] Mader TH, Carroll RD, Slade CS, et al. Ocular war injuries of the Iraqi insurgency, January–September 2004. Ophthalmology 2006;113:97–104.

[2] Gondusky JS, Reiter MP. Protecting military convoys in Iraq: an examination of battle injuries sustained by a mechanized battalion during Operation Iraqi Freedom II. Mil Med 2005;170:546–9.

[3] Xydakis MS, Fravell MD, Nasser KE, et al. Analysis of battlefield head and neck injuries in Iraq and Afghanistan. Otolaryngol Head Neck Surg 2005;133:497–504.

[4] Holcomb JB, Stansbury LG, Champion HR, et al. Understanding combat casualty care statistics. J Trauma 2006;60:397–401.

[5] Marshall TJ Jr. Combat casualty care: the Alpha Surgical Company experience during Operation Iraqi Freedom. Mil Med 2005;170:469–72.

[6] Patel TH, Wenner KA, Price SA, et al. A U.S. Army Forward Surgical Team's experience in Operation Iraqi Freedom. J Trauma 2004;57:201–7.

[7] Wedmore I, McManus JG, Pusateri AE, et al. A special report on the chitosan-based hemostatic dressing: experience in current combat operations. J Trauma 2006;60:655–8.

[8] Pusateri AE, Holcomb JB, Kheirabadi BS, et al. Making sense of the preclinical literature on advanced hemostatic products. J Trauma 2006;60:674–82.

[9] Alam HB, Burris D, DaCorta JA, et al. Hemorrhage control in the battlefield: role of new hemostatic agents. Mil Med 2005;170:63–9.

[10] Walters TJ, Mabry RL. Issues related to the use of tourniquets on the battlefield. Mil Med 2005;170:770–5.

[11] Alam HB, Koustova E, Rhee P. Combat casualty care research: from bench to the battlefield. World J Surg 2005;29(Suppl 1):S7–11.

[12] Neuffer MC, McDivitt J, Rose D, et al. Hemostatic dressings for the first responder: a review. Mil Med 2004;169:716–20.

[13] Basbaum AI. Spinal mechanisms of acute and persistent pain. Reg Anesth Pain Med 1999;24:59–67.

[14] Beilin B, Shavit Y, Trabekin E, et al. The effects of postoperative pain management on immune response to surgery. Anesth Analg 2003;97:822–7.

[15] Kotwal RS, O'Connor KC, Johnson TR, et al. A novel pain management strategy for combat casualty care. Ann Emerg Med 2004;44:121–7.

[16] Stevens RA, Bohman HR, Baker BC, et al. The U.S. Navy's forward resuscitative surgery system during Operation Iraqi Freedom. Mil Med 2005;170:297–301.

[17] Chambers LW, Rhee P, Baker BC, et al. Initial experience of US Marine Corps forward resuscitative surgical system during Operation Iraqi Freedom. Arch Surg 2005;140:26–32.

[18] Murray CK, Reynolds JC, Schroeder JM, et al. Spectrum of care provided at an echelon II Medical Unit during Operation Iraqi Freedom. Mil Med 2005;170:516–20.

[19] Szpisjak DF, Lamb CL, Klions KD. Oxygen consumption with mechanical ventilation in a field anesthesia machine. Anesth Analg 2005;100:1713–7.

[20] Lunn DV, Young PC. The Ohmeda Universal PAC drawover apparatus. A technical and clinical evaluation. Anaesthesia 1995;50:870–4.

[21] Khaing TT, Yu S, Brock-Utne JG. Inspired oxygen concentrations with or without an oxygen economizer during ether draw-over anaesthesia. Anaesth Intensive Care 1997;25:417–9.

[22] Fritz LA, Kay JK, Garrett N. Description of the oxygen concentration delivered using different combinations of oxygen reservoir volumes and supplemental oxygen flow rates

with the Ohmeda Universal Portable Anesthesia Complete draw-over vaporizer system. Mil Med 2003;168:304–11.

[23] Jarvis DA, Brock-Utne JG. Use of an oxygen concentrator linked to a draw-over vaporizer (anesthesia delivery system for underdeveloped nations). Anesth Analg 1991;72:805–10.

[24] Pylman ML, Teiken PJ. Sevoflurane concentration available from the universal drawover vaporizer. Mil Med 1997;162:405–6.

[25] Hawkins JK, Ciresi SA, Phillips WJ. Performance of the universal portable anesthesia complete vaporizer with mechanical ventilation in both drawover and pushover configurations. Mil Med 1998;163:159–63.

[26] Hawkins JK, Ciresi SA, Phillips WJ. Clinical evaluation of pushover mechanical ventilation with the Ohmeda Universal Portable Anesthesia Complete vaporizer. Mil Med 1998;163: 164–8.

[27] Paine GF, Bonnema CL, Stambaugh TA, et al. Anesthesia services aboard USNS COM-FORT (T-AH-20) during Operation Iraqi Freedom. Mil Med 2005;170:476–82.

[28] Brooks AJ, Price V, Simms M. FAST on operational military deployment. Emerg Med J 2005;22:263–5.

[29] Chambers LW. The experience of the US Marine Corps' Surgical Shock Trauma Platoon with 417 operative combat casualties during a 12-month period of Operation Iraqi Freedom. Presented at the American Association for the Surgery of Trauma Meeting. Atlanta, 2005.

[30] Fox CJ, Gillespie DL, O'Donnell SD, et al. Contemporary management of wartime vascular trauma. J Vasc Surg 2005;41:638–44.

[31] Buckenmaier CC 3rd, Lee EH, Shields CH, et al. Regional anesthesia in austere environments. Reg Anesth Pain Med 2003;28:321–7.

[32] Buckenmaier CC, McKnight GM, Winkley JV, et al. Continuous peripheral nerve block for battlefield anesthesia and evacuation. Reg Anesth Pain Med 2005;30:202–5.

ELSEVIER
SAUNDERS

Anesthesiology Clin
25 (2007) 147–160

ANESTHESIOLOGY
CLINICS

Mechanisms of Injury by Explosive Devices

Major Jeff Garner, MB ChB, MRCS(Ed), RAMC[a]
Stephen J. Brett, MD, FRCA[b],*

[a]Northern General Hospital, Herries Road, Sheffield, S5 7AU, UK
[b]Department of Anaesthesia and Intensive Care, Hammersmith Hospital,
Du Cane Road, London, W12 0HS, UK

Pathophysiology of blast injury

The understanding and management of blast injury has traditionally been the preserve of the military physician; apart from those in Northern Ireland and Israel, few civilians had any experience in blast injury; the context has now changed with the recent globalization of terrorism and it has now become necessary for nonmilitary clinicians everywhere to understand the events that generate blast injury and the ways in which the victim of a blast is injured.

Blast injury has traditionally been subdivided into four categories depending on the mechanism of injury production (Table 1), and this chapter concentrates on primary blast injury because it is the phenomenon that is most alien to doctors, whereas many of the soft tissue and penetrating fragment injuries encountered as secondary and tertiary effects will be more familiar and require less explanation.

The physics of explosions

Explosives release their energy in the form of high-pressure shock waves in a very short space of time by the process of detonation, which breaks down the chemical bonds within the explosive. A pressure wave is generated that propagates through the explosive until it reaches the explosive–air interface, where it generates a shock (blast) wave in the surrounding air and compresses a rim of air around the ball of explosive products that expands

* Corresponding author.
  E-mail address: stephen.brett@imperial.ac.uk (S.J. Brett).

0889-8537/07/$ - see front matter © 2007 Elsevier Inc. All rights reserved.
doi:10.1016/j.anclin.2006.11.002   *anesthesiology.theclinics.com*

Table 1
The four types of blast injury

Type	Mechanism of injury
Primary	Interaction of the blast wave with the body.
Secondary	Energized fragments from the explosion or debris accelerated by the blast wind.
Tertiary	Physical displacement of the body by the blast wind including tumbling; crush injury.
Quaternary	All other effects; includes the psychologic effects and burns.

rapidly. As the gases expand, they rapidly cool and slow down, and the rim of compressed air containing the pressure pulse that had been attached to the expanding ball of gaseous products detaches and propagates through the atmosphere alone. Classically, the pressure changes of the blast wave are described at a single point over time. There is a virtually instantaneous sharp rise in pressure within the air surrounding the blast rapidly attaining its *peak (static) overpressure.* As the blast wave propagates through the surrounding atmosphere, the magnitude of the pressure wave falls away in inverse proportion to the third power of the radius of its sphere of expansion. Overexpansion, because of an inertial effect in air, is followed by rarefaction and pressures below ambient pressure (*the underpressure*), which then return to ambient atmospheric pressure (Fig. 1). This classical waveform is known as a Friedlander wave and describes the pressure changes for a simple blast wave in a free field environment, ie, one without obstacles or constraints.

Passage of the blast wave not only alters the air pressure, it accelerates the air it traverses, and the mass movement of air is known as the blast wind or *dynamic overpressure.*

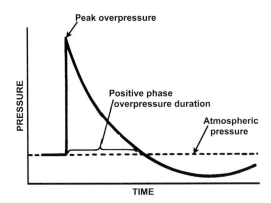

Fig. 1. Representation of the pressure at a fixed point over time as a Friedlander blast wave passes. (*From* Horrocks CL. Blast injuries: biophysics, pathophysiology and management principles. J R Army Med Corps 2001;147(1):28–40; with permission.)

Primary blast injury

In simple terms, at an interface of two materials of differing densities, a shock wave is both *reflected* and *coupled* into the incident target, and the primary blast injury is the effect of the blast wave at the air–body interface. Its effects are most noticeable where the density differential is most marked—at tissue–air junctions such as the ear, lung, and intestines. There is a short-duration, high-amplitude stress wave that propagates through the body, depositing energy at internal tissue interfaces. Long-duration shear waves cause gross deformation of the body wall with tearing of organs at points of fixed attachments.

Physiologic responses to blast waves

Thoracic blast exposure results in a reflex triad of apnea, bradycardia, and hypotension [1], probably mediated via the vagus nerve. The apnea occurs within 2 seconds of blast exposure and is usually of only a few seconds duration. The onset of bradycardia occurs a few seconds later, is maximal at 10 seconds, and effects may continue for up to an hour [2]. The hypotension is again almost immediate [2], with some recovery over time, but normotension is not achieved. Despite low systemic vascular resistance, compensatory peripheral vasoconstriction is absent, suggesting interference with cardiovascular responsiveness [3]. This triad is absent in abdominal blast exposure [4].

Blast lung

Upper respiratory tract damage may serve as an indicator of primary blast injury elsewhere [5] with bruising of the airway mucosa often corresponding to the cartilaginous rings of the trachea [6]. In the lungs proper, the stress wave's energy tears the interalveolar septa causing hemorrhage into the alveoli and bronchioles. At postmortem examination a spectrum of severity is noted from scattered small petechial hemorrhages to large areas of confluent hemorrhage—if the blast load has been particularly severe then tears of the parenchyma are apparent. Damage is greatest in areas of concentration of the stress wave such as the costophrenic angles [6] adjacent to the mediastinum (Fig. 2) [7] and the intercostal spaces (Fig. 3), which produces the striped appearance erroneously referred to as *rib markings*. Tearing of superficial alveoli and pleura gives rise to pneumothoraces, and if there is underlying parenchymal damage, hemothoraces too.

Separation of the capillaries from their supporting connective tissue creates perivascular spaces, which fill with blood, appearing as "ring haemorrhages" on light microscopy. The formation of traumatic alveolar–venous fistulae is common and results in air emboli, which contribute to the extrapulmonary pathology of primary blast injury (PBI) [6]. Ultrastructurally there is increased blebbing of the epithelial cell membrane and increased

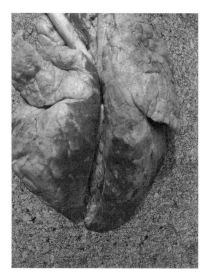

Fig. 2. Primary blast injury to the lungs. Hemorrhagic injury is most noticeable in the section of lungs that abut the mediastinum.

pinocytosis—features commonly found in the early stages of lung trauma of other etiologies [8]. These changes were evident in macroscopically normal and microscopically minimally injured lungs 30 minutes after blast exposure and changed over time. Twenty-four hours after blast, there was macroscopic evidence of hemorrhage in the previously unmarked lung from the side not directly exposed to blast, and the ultrastructural changes were more widespread than at 30 minutes after injury, suggesting that the development of primary blast lung injury is a dynamic process that continues after passage of the blast wave.

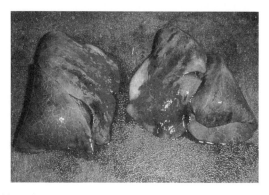

Fig. 3. "Rib markings" in pulmonary primary blast injury. (*From* Horrocks CL. Blast injuries: biophysics, pathophysiology and management principles. J R Army Med Corps 2001;147(1): 28–40; with permission.)

The macro- and microscopic injuries outlined present clinically with a well recognized but nonspecific constellation of signs and symptoms. Dyspnea and a cough are usual—the cough is initially dry but progresses to produce frothy sputum and, later, hemoptysis; hemoptysis may occasionally be overwhelming and immediately life-threatening. Chest pain is typically retrosternal. Examination finds tachypnea and cyanosis, dullness to percussion, decreased breath sounds, and widespread coarse rhonchi. Hemo-/pneumothorax and subcutaneous emphysema may be evident. Retrosternal emphysema is indicative of pneumomediastinum. Inspection of the optic fundi may disclose air emboli suggesting pulmonary injury. The blood-filled alveoli limit gas exchange, and a marked shunt is evident with the patient becoming progressively hypoxic and hypocarbic [9]. The chest x-ray shows typical bilateral butterfly wing infiltrates [10] that become maximal by 48 hours and then resolve over the following few days. Persistent infiltrates suggest the development of acute respiratory distress syndrome or pneumonia. Most cases of blast lung are apparent on admission to the hospital [11], although some investigators contend that symptoms may develop up to 48 hours after exposure [12].

Cardiac blast injury

Although occasional cases of direct cardiac damage from blast loading are reported, the majority of blast-related cardiac pathology and immediate PBI deaths are from air emboli within the coronary circulation [13], although the experimental evidence is limited [4]. Coronary emboli may provoke arrhythmias, ischemia, or frank myocardial infarction.

Abdominal blast injury

The different effects of long- and short-duration blast waves are more easily discernible in the abdomen. Coupled short-duration stress waves deposit energy at the mucosal surface of the small intestine in a similar manner to alveolar wall disruption—higher overpressures cause direct small bowel perforation, whereas lesser overpressures generate mural contusions that spread from mucosa to serosa [14] and are at risk of delayed perforation up to 2 weeks after injury. The solid abdominal organs, retroperitoneal colon, and small bowel mesentery appear to be injured by the long-duration shear waves generated by the gross displacement of the abdominal wall (Fig. 4). At laparotomy for abdominal blast injury, there may be multiple contusions potentially requiring extensive bowel resection to obviate the risk of later perforation. Animal studies have now defined those contusions at high risk of delayed perforation and thus warranting resection: small bowel contusions ≥15 mm in diameter, those occupying more than half the bowel circumference or sited on the antemesenteric border, and colonic contusions ≥20 mm diameter [15]. Abdominal blast injury is relatively more common in underwater blasts [16].

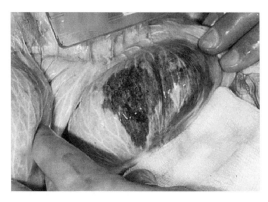

Fig. 4. Primary blast injury to the colon. (*From* Horrocks CL. Blast injuries: biophysics, pathophysiology and management principles. J R Army Med Corps 2001;147(1):28–40; with permission.)

Auditory blast injury

The tympanic membrane will rupture at overpressures as low as 35 kPa, and half will have ruptured by the time the overpressure reaches 104 kPa [17], but it correlates poorly with blast injury elsewhere and is of no use as a predictive marker. Leibovici and colleagues [11] report nearly 650 survivors of explosion exposure, 193 of whom had evidence of blast injury. Three quarters had isolated eardrum rupture—none subsequently had other blast injuries, whereas nearly 10% of cases had pulmonary blast injury with intact tympanic membranes. The ossicular chain may also be disrupted by the blast injury. Sensineural deafness and tinnitus are frequent accompaniments to blast exposure—they often resolve spontaneously within a few hours, but the incidence of permanent hearing loss by blast exposure is as high as 55% [18]. Of interest in auditory blast injury is an incidence of 12% of subsequent cholesteatoma development after implantation of squamous keratinizing epithelium into the middle ear after perforation of the tympanic membrane [19], the incidence being related to the degree of perforation [20].

Orthopedic primary blast injury

Traumatic amputation after blast exposure is not a result of flailing and avulsion as previously thought, but mostly occurs through the long bone shafts with only 1 of 56 lower limb traumatic amputations occurring through a joint [21]. Experimental evidence has shown that stress wave passing close to a long bone couples energy into the bone causing bone failure [22]. Sites of predilection are the upper third of tibia and upper and lower thirds of the femur in the lower limb and the proximal thirds of both arm and forearm. After fracture it is the following dynamic overpressure that separates the fractured extremity. Traumatic amputation or partial amputation not obviously caused by a large secondary fragment is rare in survivors [23] and is a potential marker of severe blast exposure.

Secondary blast injury

Secondary blast injury is by penetration of energized missiles. The injury produced is a function of the energy transferred to the target, itself dependent on the available energy and the retardation to the missile offered by the incident tissue. Penetrating missiles create a wound track by direct laceration and a radial displacement of the surrounding tissues by temporary cavitation—the cavity is at subatmospheric pressure and may suck in external contaminants. One of the determining factors in the degree of clinical injury in penetrating fragment trauma is the degree to which the tissues can accept the cavitation—elastic tissues such as lung suffer little permanent damage, whereas denser tissues such as liver within its fibrous capsule accept cavitation poorly and shatter. Thus, the primary determinants of the impact of secondary blast injury are the level of energy transfer, the sensitivity of the injured tissues, and the extent and nature of contamination [24]. In most intentional explosions, secondary blast effects predominate. The intensity of the blast wave diminishes rapidly as its radius increases, but the energized fragments retain sufficient kinetic energy for penetration for a much greater distance. This explains the observation that primary blast injury is rare in survivors of explosions but much more common in those killed outright—in essence, victims close enough to the source of explosion to suffer PBI are usually overwhelmed by the secondary (and tertiary) blast effects [25]. An interesting development in terrorist bombings is the potential for the transfer of infectious diseases from implantation of biological remnants from suicide bombers. Three cases of suicide bomb survivors being penetrated by bone shards of the perpetrators have been reported, one of which was Hepatitis B positive although the victim was not infected [26].

Tertiary blast injury

These are effects from the bodily displacement of the victim and are largely a consequence of the dynamic overpressure. Traumatic amputation is a combination of primary and tertiary effects and is extremely rare in survivors of blast exposure; Fykberg and Tepas [23] report an incidence of traumatic amputation of 1.2% in a series of nearly 3000 immediate survivors of blast exposure. In long-duration blast waves such as those produced by nuclear detonations, blast wind effects predominate over the blast overpressure. Blast winds may achieve speeds of up to 160 km/h and human fatalities from tumbling induced by the blast wind start at wind speeds of 80 km/h; ground impact speeds of 35 km/h are sufficient to kill half of those so affected [27]. It is estimated that 70% of survivors of the atomic detonations at Hiroshima and Nagasaki suffered injury from either flying debris or being bodily displaced [28]. Crush injury—another tertiary effect—may also contribute significantly to the death and injury toll from bomb explosions [29].

Quaternary blast effects

This diverse group includes all other sequelae of blast exposure. The two most commonly seen quaternary effects are psychological problems, which may be significant in both survivors and nonexposed individuals [30], and burns. Although explosions generate an enormous amount of thermal energy, it is short lived, and burns are superficial from radiant heat; the exposed skin (hands, arms, and face) are the areas affected.

Special situations

The discussion so far has described blast in an unrestrained free-field environment, but clearly not all explosions occur in such idealized circumstances; explosions in areas in which complex waves are formed increase the destructive power.

Enhanced blast weapons

Enhanced blast weapons deliberately use the blast wave to engage the target by detonation of a liquid hydrocarbon dispersed throughout the atmosphere. The vapor cloud detonates generating a blast wave of lower peak overpressure than a comparable mass of conventional explosive but one that covers a far greater area, maintains its peak overpressure for longer, and decays in intensity at the periphery of the cloud more slowly (Fig. 5). There are little in the way of secondary blast effects. They are particularly effective against field defenses and buildings and have been used in Afghanistan, Chechnya [31], and Iraq [28].

Enclosed spaces

Explosions in enclosed spaces, or external blasts that enter an enclosed space, are designated complex waves and behave differently from Friedlander waves. The walls of the enclosure act as reflecting surfaces with the reflected blast wave combining with the incident wave to increase the magnitude of the associated overpressure. Detonations at the junction of two walls or in a corner increase the effective yield by up to 4 or 8 times. Enclosures with vents such as windows or doors discharge some of the pressure wave through these vents, generating a free-field wave outside; conversely

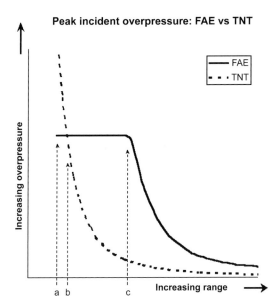

Fig. 5. The overpressure curves for 1 kg of conventional high explosive (TNT) and 1 kg of a fuel-air explosive. (*From* Horrocks CL. Blast injuries: biophysics, pathophysiology and management principles. J R Army Med Corps 2001;147(1):28–40; with permission.)

a Friedlander wave entering an enclosure through vents will subsequently reflect to form complex waves of greater peak overpressure than the external classical wave. The complex additive nature of blast within confined spaces is reflected in the number and site of casualties and fatalities that are concentrated at the sites of blast reflection [32]. In a terrorist bus bombing there was a high incidence of primary blast injury (11 lung, 4 abdominal), but some passengers adjacent to the bomb were unharmed while many of the injured were seated on the opposite side of the bus beyond the lethal radius of secondary missiles [33]. Leibovici and colleagues [34] compared two open air bombings with two bus bombings. The size and composition of the devices and density of surrounding people were thought to be similar, yet there was a highly significant increase in mortality and incidence of primary blast injury from confined bombings. The bus bombings took place in winter, and the investigators suggest that because all the vehicle's windows were closed, no venting occurred, and in the few milliseconds for which the bus's structure remained intact, the occupants would have been exposed to a massively increased static overpressure.

Blast underwater

Underwater explosions initially mirror a free air detonation with shock wave generation and an expanding sphere of gaseous products. Water is a more efficient transmission medium than air, and the effective lethal radius of the blast wave triples. Conversely, there is a greater retardation of fragments so the lethal radius of the secondary blast effects is reduced. The mass movement of water also causes a water ram effect generating gross body wall distortion, initiating intracorporeal shear waves—injuries such as hepatic lacerations from gall bladder avulsion may occur [35]. The surface air–/water interface reflects the incident pressure wave, and the complex wave produced has a reductive rather than additive effect with reduced lethality nearer the surface. An underwater blast is associated with an increased incidence of abdominal blast injury—thoracic blast injury is reduced because the chest is often out of the water, and because blast effects increase with depth, the submerged abdomen is most liable to injury: of 32 survivors of an underwater explosion during the Arab–Israeli war of 1967, all but one had primary blast injury: 27 had pulmonary blast injury, and 22 had gastrointestinal perforations at laparotomy [36]. Similarly, Gordon-Taylor [37] describes seven of 24 sailors exposed to underwater blast suffering gastrointestinal perforation. The evidence suggests that if an underwater blast is expected, then floating on your back on the surface is the safest position.

Landmines

Despite a ban on landmine usage, approximately 70 million mines still lie in unmarked minefields in 70 countries throughout the world [38]. Twenty-four thousand new deaths or injuries are reported annually from landmines [39]. Detonation releases the shock wave, hot gaseous products of explosion, the blast wind, and fragments akin to a standard explosion. The shock wave is coupled into the limb and leads to microvascular injury, soft tissue stripping, and stress fractures of the long bones [22]. Its effects may be discernible as proximal as the upper thigh, and demyelination of peripheral nerves may occur for up to 30 cm above the level of gross tissue injury [40]. Over the short distances involved, the flow of energized gaseous products strips and erodes soft tissues and induces substantial torsion and bending stresses on the limb, which may already have been fractured by the shock wave. The dynamic overpressure may detach the limb at the site of fracture. Both the flow of gaseous products and the blast wind serve to implant environmental debris, small fragments of mine case, soil, and destroyed footwear for a significant distance up the injured limb, infiltrating along the tissue planes separated by the shock wave and gaseous products and contaminating the limb beyond the level of visible destruction. The upward flow of fragments also constitutes a threat to ocular integrity—4.5% of all landmine injuries in Afghanistan were to the eyes, and two thirds were penetrating trauma [40].

The combination of these mechanisms affects gross destruction of the lower limb, which may require amputation at a high level to gain uncontaminated soft tissue coverage. The contralateral limb is usually less severely affected, although soft tissue damage and contamination from penetrating debris do occur.

Blast through armor

Personal body armor is designed to limit the effect of penetrating missiles and undoubtedly reduces the incidence of secondary injury in blast-exposed individuals; however, there is evidence that it may compound the primary effects of a blast. British Army data from Northern Ireland show a higher incidence of primary blast injury in fatally injured soldiers—90% of whom were wearing body armor, compared with "unprotected" civilians. It is proposed that wearing protection against fragment injury allowed soldiers closer to the center of the explosion, exposing them to a greater degree of primary blast [25]. Experimental findings also suggest body armor increases the intrathoracic blast pressure. Human volunteers exposed to a simulated artillery muzzle blast wearing Kevlar cloth ballistic protection vests resulted in an increased intrathoracic pressure compared with volunteers dressed in ordinary clothing [41]. An animal study using higher levels of blast loading confirmed that Kevlar vests increased lung injury in those exposed to a moderate blast overpressure and mortality in those exposed to a severe blast loading, although there was no difference in lung weights in the severe blast loading group and no clear difference in measured intrathoracic pressure in any group [42]. Potentially, the vests may increase presented thoracic area and thus increase the total blast loading, or the Kevlar may alter the impedance interfaces, such that coupling is increased. Currently, the threat from penetrating ballistic injury significantly outweighs that from primary blast effects and the use of antifragment body armor should continue.

The effects of a blast within an armored fighting vehicle (AFV) are rarely reported, as the principal threat within a penetrated AFV has been fragment injury. Improvements in design and materials have now significantly reduced this threat, suggesting that blast injury may now become a more frequent concern, although the evidence for this is scarce. Reports from the Arab–Israeli war suggested that many casualties injured within AFVs penetrated by antitank-guided missiles (ATGM) suffered burns and pulmonary injury ascribed to a combination of inhalation of toxic smoke and pulmonary PBI—described as the ATGM syndrome [43]. Since then, there have been few data to verify these effects—animals placed within AFVs but outside of the zone of fragmentation injury showed no evidence of blast injury when the vehicles were penetrated by a variety of missiles [44]. It does seem likely, however, that penetration of armor will generate some degree of blast injury, although its contribution to the overall clinical picture is unclear.

Summary

Exposure to the effects of explosions is increasingly common, and the management of the injuries produced is no longer the sole domain of the military doctor. Explosions generate thermal energy, a cloud of expanding gaseous products and a shock wave that propagates through the atmosphere. In the open, the magnitude of the pressure wave decreases far more rapidly than the dispersal of fragments energized by both the flow of explosive products and the mass movement of the air from the passage of the shock wave. Fragment injuries predominate in most circumstances, but injury from the coupling of the blast wave into the body does occur, and in certain situations—explosions underwater and in enclosed spaces— primary blast injury may predominate. The injuries of primary blast injury occur mainly at tissue density interfaces, and the small intestine, lung, and ear are particularly at risk. Transmission of the shock waves energy at these interfaces damages the tissues and generates reproducible patterns of injury. In patients exposed to an explosion, blast injury should be considered a potential contributor to mortality and morbidity.

References

[1] Guy RJ, Kirkman E, Watkins PE, et al. Physiologic responses to primary blast. J Trauma 1998;45(6):983–7.
[2] Ohnishi M, Kirkman E, Guy RJ, et al. Reflex nature of the cardiorespiratory response to primary thoracic blast injury in the anaesthetised rat. Exp Physiol 2001;86(3):357–64.
[3] Irwin RJ, Lerner MR, Bealer JF, et al. Cardiopulmonary physiology of primary blast injury. J Trauma 1997;43(4):650–5.
[4] Guy RJ, Watkins PE, Edmondstone WM. Electrocardiographic changes following primary blast injury to the thorax. J R Nav Med Serv 2000;86(3):125–33.
[5] Dodd KT, Yelverton JT, Richmond DR, et al. Nonauditory injury threshold for repeated intense freefield impulse noise. J Occup Med 1990;32(3):260–6.
[6] Chiffelle TL. Pathology of direct air blast injury. *Technical progress report on contract DA-49-146-XZ-055 Ref No DASA-1778*. Albuquerque (NM): Lovelace Foundation for Medeical Education and Research; 1966.
[7] Cooper GJ, Taylor DE. Biophysics of impact injury to the chest and abdomen. J R Army Med Corps 1989;135(2):58–67.
[8] Brown RF, Cooper GJ, Maynard RL. The ultrastructure of rat lung following acute primary blast injury. Int J Exp Pathol 1993;74(2):151–62.
[9] Mellor SG. The pathogenesis of blast injury and its management. Br J Hosp Med 1988;39(6): 536–9.
[10] Pizov R, Oppenheim-Eden A, Matot I, et al. Blast lung injury from an explosion on a civilian bus. Chest 1999;115(1):165–72.
[11] Leibovici D, Gofrit ON, Shapira SC. Eardrum perforation in explosion survivors: is it a marker of pulmonary blast injury? Ann Emerg Med 1999;34(2):168–72.
[12] Coppel DL. Blast injuries of the lungs. Br J Surg 1976;63(10):735–7.
[13] Clemedson CJ, Hultman HI. Air embolism and the cause of death in blast injury. Mil Surg 1954;114(6):424–37.
[14] Goligher JC, King DP, Simmons HT. Injuries produced by blast in water. Lancet 1943;2: 119–23.
[15] Cripps NP, Cooper GJ. Risk of late perforation in intestinal contusions caused by explosive blast. Br J Surg 1997;84(9):1298–303.
[16] Rawlins JS. Physical and pathophysiological effects of blast. Injury 1978;9(4):313–20.
[17] Kerr AG. Blast injuries to the ear. Practitioner 1978;221:677–82.

[18] Chandler DW, Edmond CV. Effects of blast overpressure on the ear: case reports. J Am Acad Audiol 1997;8:81–8.

[19] Seaman RW, Newell RC. Another etiology of middle ear cholesteatoma. Arch Otolaryngol 1971;94(5):440–2.

[20] Kronenberg J, Ben-Shoshan J, Modan M, et al. Blast injury and cholesteatoma. Am J Otol 1988;9:127–30.

[21] Hull JB, Bowyer GW, Cooper GJ, et al. Pattern of injury in those dying from traumatic amputation caused by bomb blast. Br J Surg 1994;81(8):1132–5.

[22] Hull JB, Cooper GJ. Pattern and mechanism of traumatic amputation by explosive blast. J Trauma 1996;40(3 Suppl):S198–205.

[23] Frykberg ER, Tepas JJ 3rd. Terrorist bombings. Lessons learned from Belfast to Beirut. Ann Surg 1988;208(5):569–76.

[24] Hill PF, Edwards DP, Bowyer GW. Small fragment wounds: biophysics, pathophysiology and principles of management. J R Army Med Corps 2001;147:41–51.

[25] Mellor SG, Cooper GJ. Analysis of 828 servicemen killed or injured by explosion in Northern Ireland 1970–84: the Hostile Action Casualty System. Br J Surg 1989;76(10):1006–10.

[26] Eshkol Z, Katz K. Injuries from biologic material of suicide bombers. Injury 2005;36(2): 271–4.

[27] Bellamy RF, Zajtchuk R. The weapons of conventional land warfare. In: Bellamy RF, Zajtchuk R, editors. Textbook of military medicine part 1, vol. 2, Medical consequences of nuclear warfare. Washington, DC: US Government printing Office; 1989. p. 4–5.

[28] Ripple GR, Phillips Y, et al. Military explosions. In: Cooper GJ, Dudley HAF, Gann SF, editors. Scientific foundations of trauma. Oxford (UK): Butterworth-Heinemann; 1997. p. 247–57.

[29] Mellor SG, et al. Terrorist bombings: patterns of injury. In: Cooper GJ, Dudley HAF, Gann SF, editors. Scientific foundations of trauma. Oxford (UK): Butterworth-Heinemann; 1997. p. 236–46.

[30] Tucker P, Pfefferbaum B, Vincent R, et al. Oklahoma city: disaster challenges mental health and medical administrators. J Behav Health Serv Res 1998;25(1):93–9.

[31] Phillips YY, Richmond DR. Primary blast injury and basic research: a brief history. In: Bellamy RF, Zajtchuk R, editors. Textbook of military medicine, part 1, vol. 1, Conventional warfare: ballistic, blast and burn injuries. Washington, DC: US Government Printing Office; 1990. p. 227–33.

[32] Cooper GJ, Maynard RL, Cross NL, et al. Casualties from terrorist bombings. J Trauma 1983;23(11):955–67.

[33] Katz E, Ofek B, Adler J, et al. Primary blast injury after a bomb explosion in a civilian bus. Ann Surg 1989;209(4):484–8.

[34] Leibovici D, Gofrit ON, Stein M, et al. Blast injuries: bus versus open-air bombings—a comparative study of injuries in survivors of open-air versus confined-space explosions. J Trauma 1996;41(6):1030–5.

[35] Cooper GJ, Jönsson A, et al. Protection against blast injury. In: Cooper GJ, Dudley HAF, Gann SF, editors. Scientific foundations of trauma. Oxford (UK): Butterworth-Heinemann; 1997. p. 258–83.

[36] Huller T, Bazini Y. Blast injuries of the chest and abdomen. Arch Surg 1970;100(1):24–30.

[37] Gordon-Taylor G. Abdominal effects of immersion blast. In: Cope Z, editor. Surgery, part 2. London: HMSO; 1953. p. 664–72.

[38] Wennerstrom M, Baaser S, Salama P, et al. Injuries associated with landmines and unexploded ordnance—Afghanistan, 1997–2002. Morb Mortal Wkly Rep 2003;52(36):859–62.

[39] Giannou C. Antipersonnel landmines: facts, fictions, and priorities. BMJ 1997;315:1453–4.

[40] Trimble K, Clasper J. Anti-personnel mine injury; mechanism and medical management. J R Army Med Corps 2001;147(1):73–9.

[41] Young AJ, Jaeger JJ, Phillips YY, et al. The influence of clothing on human intrathoracic pressure during airblast. Aviat Space Environ Med 1985;56(1):49–53.

[42] Phillips YY, Mundie TG, Yelverton JT, et al. Cloth ballistic vest alters response to blast. J Trauma 1988;28(1 Suppl):S149–52.

[43] Owen-Smith M. Armoured fighting vehicle casualties. J R Army Med Corps 1977;123:65–76.

[44] Phillips YY, Mundie TG, Hoyt R, et al. Middle ear injury in animals exposed to complex blast waves inside an armored vehicle. Ann Otol Rhinol Laryngol Suppl 1989;140:17–22.

ELSEVIER
SAUNDERS

Anesthesiology Clin
25 (2007) 161–177

ANESTHESIOLOGY
CLINICS

Disaster Preparedness, Triage, and Surge Capacity for Hospital Definitive Care Areas: Optimizing Outcomes when Demands Exceed Resources

J. David Roccaforte, MD[a,b,*], James G. Cushman, MD[c]

[a]Department of Anesthesiology, New York University, New York, NY, USA
[b]Department of Anesthesia, Bellevue Hospital, Room 11N34, First Ave. at 27th St.,
New York, NY 10016, USA
[c]Department of Surgery, University of Maryland, R. Adams Cowley Shock Trauma Center,
22 South Greene St., Baltimore, MD 21201, USA

Disaster planning must anticipate how demands imposed by a disaster reconcile with the capacity of the treating facility. Resources must be organized before an event such that they are optimally used to treat as many victims as possible, as well as to avoid overwhelming available resources. Hirshberg and colleagues [1] in 2001 defined two different scenarios based on this supply–demand relationship. By their definitions, the absolute numbers of victims are less relevant than how demands reconcile with the capacity of the receiving facility. Multiple casualty incidents (MCIs) are defined as a large number of casualties generated over a short period that are appropriately managed with existing or extended resources. Mass casualty events (MCEs) in contrast, are major medical disasters that erode organized community support mechanisms and result in casualties which overwhelm resources.

Following the September 11, 2001, attack in Lower Manhattan, several hospitals reported the volume and pattern of injuries they treated [2–4]. Consistent with existing literature describing explosive terrorist events (especially involving a building collapse), most of the victims died at the scene, there were few casualties (relative to the number killed), and even fewer critically injured patients who survived to hospitalization [5–10].

* Corresponding author. Department of Anesthesia, Bellevue Hospital, Room 11N34, First Ave. at 27th St., New York, NY 10016.
  E-mail address: jdavidr@mail.com (J.D. Roccaforte).

Analysis of all casualties reported from the three main Lower Manhattan receiving hospitals on the morning of September 11, 2001, shows that no hospital was overwhelmed by critically injured patients. Further analysis of casualty data comparing New York University–Downtown Hospital (NYU-DH) with Bellevue Hospital (BH) shows a linear association between critical mortality and overtriage, consistent with the findings of Frykberg [7].

The subsequent discussion analyzes the concept of surge capacity and reviews relevant characteristics of disaster events, victims of such events, and hospital resources. The dilemma of triage for definitive care areas (DCAs) such as operating rooms (ORs) and intensive care units (ICUs) is also presented, along with the relevant victim characteristics. Lastly, using tabletop exercises, the discussion addresses what can be done pre-event to prepare a DCA for a multiple or mass casualty event.

Lower Manhattan casualty data from September 11, 2001

On the morning of September 11, 2001, organizers of the BH surgical response recorded 169 casualties. Approximately half of the casualties were uninjured (requiring no medical evaluation beyond triage and first aid). Of patients further evaluated, only a minority required comprehensive surgical management. Table 1 includes casualty data for BH on September 11th and the following 6 days.

Table 2 summarizes the cumulative casualty data from the three Manhattan hospitals located below 42nd Street: two state-designated level 1 trauma centers (BH and St. Vincent's Medical Center), and one university-affiliated community hospital (NYU-DH).

A total of 1755 patients were evaluated at these three facilities during the first week. Fully 90% of patients arriving required no formal medical evaluation beyond triage and registration. For this reason, Lower Manhattan hospitals experienced what was essentially concurrent medical MCIs yielding primarily an exercise in crowd management and information processing (Fig. 1) [11].

The 181 patients evaluated over the first week at these hospitals represent an approximately threefold increase in volume. This increase in case volume

Table 1
September 11, 12–18, 2001, casualties received at Bellevue Hospital

Time	No. casualties received	Obviously uninjured	Patients triaged	Medical evaluation	Surgical evaluation
September 11	169	83	86	74	12
Days 2–7	25	2	23	14	9
Total	194	85	109	88	21 (19% of 109 patients triaged)

Data from Cushman JG, Pachter L, Beaton HL. Two New York City hospitals' surgical responses to the September 11, 2001, terrorist attack in New York City. J Trauma 2003;54: 147–55.

Table 2
September 11–18, 2001, casualties received at Lower Manhattan Hospitals

Hospital	Patients received	Obviously uninjured	Patients evaluated	Operations performed	Patient transfers	Deaths
BH	194	85	109	10	1	3
NYU-DH	717	691	26	8	22	7
St. Vincent's Hospital	844	798	46	NA	3	5
Total	1755	1574 (90% of 1755 received)	181 (10% requiring full evaluation)	≥18	26	15

Abbreviation: NA, not available.

Data from Cushman JG, Pachter L, Beaton HL. Two New York City hospitals' surgical response to the September 11, 2001, terrorist attack in New York City. J Trauma 2003;54: 147–55; Feeney JM, Goldberg R, Blumenthal JA, et al. September 11, 2001, revisited. Arch Surg 2005;140:1068–73.

stressed the resources only at the hospital nearest to Ground Zero (NYU-DH). To complicate matters, NYU-DH was partially disabled by simultaneous internal disasters: impaired access to the hospital, loss of electricity, and poor air quality.

Triage, overtriage, critical mortality, and definitive care areas

On October 23, 1983, a suicide truck bomb destroyed the US Marine barracks in Beirut. Lieutenant Erik Frykberg, a general surgeon, was the chief medical officer on board the USS Iwo Jima. With limited resources and staff, Dr. Frykberg managed all 112 injured survivors. The explosion generated 346 casualties, of whom 234 immediately died. Of the 112 survivors, 96 were injured. Only 19 survivors were critical, defined by an Injury Severity

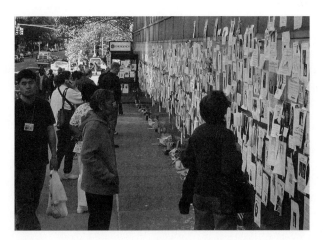

Fig. 1. Fliers posted in New York City requesting information regarding missing persons following the September 11, 2001, attacks. (*Courtesy of* Ken Sutin, MD, New York, NY.)

Score (ISS) of 15 or greater. The 77 lightly injured survivors (ISS < 15) created an overtriage rate (77/96) of 80%. Among the 112 initial survivors, there were 7 additional deaths, all among the 19 critically injured. Frykberg realized that the overall mortality of survivors (7/112 or 6.3%) did not tell the whole story. He concluded that a better gauge of the medical response in a disaster would be the "critical mortality," or those deaths occurring among the critically injured as a proportion of all critically injured. Because all 7 late deaths in the Beirut bombing occurred among those with an ISS greater than or equal to 15, the *critical mortality* was 7/19 or 37%, a statistic undiluted by the majority of survivors who did not have significant injury. Of note within this definition: moribund victims with nonsurvivable injuries are not counted as initial survivors.

Frykberg reviewed multiple terrorist bombing events and noted a fascinating trend. As overtriage increases, so does critical mortality ($r = 0.92$) [7,12]. The explanation for this relationship is twofold. First, sorting through numerous victims to find the few critically injured takes valuable time. Second, an excess of patients who have minor injuries or no injuries prevents the DCA from functioning optimally. Predictably, radiology becomes a bottleneck; laboratory results are lost or delayed, phone lines are overloaded, medications are not properly dispensed, charts are incomplete, and staff become stressed and tired. Consequently, although individuals working in the DCAs may be under the impression that they are providing appropriate care, all of these seemingly inconsequential inadequacies conspire to increase the mortality of those patients whose lives hang in the balance and require immediate, uncompromised definitive care for survival.

Thus, while the treatment of non–critical victims is not the direct responsibility of a DCA, the consequences of their presence significantly impairs efforts to care for the critically ill and injured. Often during a disaster, caregivers adopt a siege mentality. Consequently, the insidious distractions and delays that overtriage causes are not overtly obvious to those working in the ORs and ICUs and are virtually incomprehensible to others (eg, the local officials, hospital administrators, prehospital providers, and emergency physicians who are largely responsible for planning the management of the medical response upstream from DCAs).

Lower Manhattan critical mortality data from September 11, 2001

The relationship between overtriage and critical mortality appears to have been demonstrated again on September 11, 2001. Surgeons from NYU-DH, the facility nearest to the World Trade Center, and BH analyzed and calculated their overtriage and critical mortality rates [2]. Because of its proximity, NYU-DH was flooded with psychologic casualties, the uninjured seeking refuge, people looking for missing colleagues, and critically injured victims brought in by bystanders as well as by ambulance. At BH, many ambulatory victims also arrived for evaluation, but the critically injured were mostly transported by emergency medical services (EMS). At BH, the overtriage rate was 80%, and the critical mortality was 28%, which was similar to the Beirut bombing. At NYU-DH, overtriage was 95%, and the critical mortality was 44%, which are the highest values reported from any disaster to date.

Placing these data points from September 11, 2001, on Frykberg's graph, the linear relationship is maintained (Fig. 2).

The challenges at NYU-DH arose from both sides of the demands/resources equation: First, mainly as a consequence of victims presenting to the nearest hospital while bypassing the EMS selection process, the resulting overtriage placed excessive demands on hospital resources. Second, because of its proximity to the tower disaster, NYU-DH's critical hospital infrastructure failed, causing an internal disaster that compromised available resources.

Discussion

Surge capacity

Dr. Tara O'Toole [13], Director of the Center for Biosecurity at the University of Pittsburgh Medical Center, emphasized three key response areas related to the state of preparation for a bioterrorist attack: (1) public health system vulnerabilities (eg, limited United States laboratory capacity for processing huge volumes of specimens), (2) inability to provide adequate doses

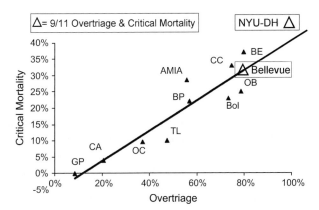

Fig. 2. Linear association between overtriage and critical mortality in selected terrorist events ($r = 0.92$ for data points). AMIA, Buenos Aires; BE, Beirut; Bol, Bologna; BP, Birmingham pubs; CA, Craigavon; CC, Cu Chi; GP, Guildford pubs; OB, Old Bailey; OC, Oklahoma City; TL, Tower of London. (*Graph adapted from* Frykberg ER. Medical management of disasters and mass casualties from terrorist bombings: how can we cope? J Trauma 2002;53:208; with permission. *Data from* Cushman JG, Pachter HL, Beaton HL. Two New York City hospitals' surgical response to the September 11, 2001, terrorist attack in New York City. J Trauma 2003;54:151.)

of vaccinations and medications to treat major bioweapon agents, and (3) lack of hospital surge capacity or inability to expand services, primarily due to financial constraints. Subsequent to global terrorism on American soil, references to disaster preparedness surge capacity have increased [14].

For example, in US Senate testimony, Dr. Elaine Kamarck [15] stated, "recent trends in medicine in the U.S. have resulted in less capacity to deal with a 'surge' in demand for serious medical care than ever before...the absence of 'surge capacity' is serious when contemplating a high number of injuries resulting from a terrorist attack involving explosives; the absence becomes even more dangerous when contemplating the number needing medical care that could arise from a bioterrorist attack."

An early and clearly relevant use of the term "surge capacity" with regard to terrorist-related disaster threat was introduced by Smithson and Levy [16] in 2000. These authors reported that several cities "plan to establish a surge capacity at the hospitals, as well as medical outposts away from them." The idea of medical outposts referred to the creation of overflow capacity for temporarily managing excessive numbers of non–critically injured or ill victims at buildings other than the hospital, such as field centers, large indoor arenas, stadiums, schools, mobile field care centers, and so forth [16]. Rational and appropriate management of such noncritical casualties is an integral component to instituting surge capacity at any level; excessive casualties inappropriately triaged will have a powerful adverse effect on critical mortality outcomes.

The casualty data from the Lower Manhattan hospital response to September 11, 2001, is illustrative of several aspects of disaster preparedness. On that date, New York City was not prepared to respond to a sudden disaster that yielded nearly 2000 casualties where 90% of victims did not require the resources of the city's trauma centers. Chelsea Piers, converted to a medical outpost, was ill-designed for critically injured patients [7] and received few, if any, injured victims. It has been suggested that the United States' shortfall in medical preparedness for such a disaster has yet to be corrected [15,17].

Before disaster planning can take place, it is important to understand the relevant characteristics of disaster events (causes), casualties (victims), resources, and how they interrelate. Planning must acknowledge that the pinnacle of the medical response to any disaster takes place in definitive care areas. Thus, a critical component of disaster planning must be preservation of DCA capability and effectiveness.

Relevant characteristics of disaster events

A simple and relevant classification scheme for DCA preparation is to consider the disaster event location (internal or external) and the speed of onset (rapid or slow) (Fig. 3).

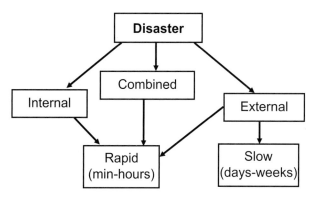

Fig. 3. Functional classification of disasters based on location and onset.

Fire [18], electrical failure [19,20], and flooding [21,22] are examples of internal disasters that affect hospital infrastructure. Examples of external disasters would include St. Vincent's Hospital and BH on September 11, 2001, or the Israeli experience in terrorist bombings [23,24]. Combined internal/external disasters present particularly difficult challenges. Examples include the NYU-DH experience on September 11th, 2001, and an earthquake occurring in an urban area [25].

Slowly evolving events include infectious epidemics [26] and hurricanes [27]. With severe acute respiratory syndrome (SARS), for example, the worldwide surge in patients peaked at 56 days following initial case reports [28]. The delay in the surge of casualties allows administrators to implement plans, adjust resources, and request and obtain outside assistance. In contrast, rapidly evolving disasters require pre-event plans, frequent drills, and a self-sufficient local response that can be rapidly mobilized. Failure to have such capabilities leaves the seriously ill or injured victims most vulnerable.

Because the scope of variation in event types is so diverse, rational planning either involves generalization in broad terms (the all hazards approach), or identification of a hypothetical list of high-risk events to guide training (the hazard vulnerability analysis approach), or a combination of the two strategies [14].

Relevant characteristics of victims and triage

While unique in proportion and precedent, the September 11, 2001, attacks were illustrative of the casualty spectrum identified in most rapidly evolving disasters [21,22]. There were victims who were immediately killed, were not immediately killed but moribund, were critically injured with the potential for survival, others who required medical evaluation but were not critical ("walking wounded"), and those who experienced psychologic effects only ("worried well").

Frykberg [7] was among the first to describe the dead/injured ratio for a variety of terrorist bombings. He observed in Beirut a dead/injured ratio of 2:1, a reversal of the 1:2 to 1:5 ratio of conventional war. Frykberg further noted that the dead/injured ratio of the September 11, 2001, attack would be 5:1 or higher, and in fact, it may have approached 10:1. In most reports from various mass casualty events, deaths and injuries can be tabulated. The dead/injured ratio is proving to be a recurring statistic that correlates to the amount of physical energy released by the event.

The American College of Surgeons [29] recommends that trauma centers maintain a 50% overtriage rate for the management of casualties from physical injury under routine circumstances; ie, half of the patients triaged to a trauma center are found not to have sustained major trauma (as defined by an ISS < 15). Thus, prehospital protocols are designed to encourage a degree of overtriage. The intent is to capture all serious injuries while minimizing the opposite result of undertriage and having seriously injured trauma patients inappropriately treated at nontrauma centers. Frykberg recognized that in disaster scenarios the dead may vastly outnumber the injured, and only a minority of those injured are critical (10%–15%), so overtriage above and beyond the 50% mark was possible, with potentially deleterious consequences to the survival of the critically injured.

In response to multiple or mass casualty, the most basic distinction is between those casualties who are critical versus noncritical. As one follows the path of the victim from the scene, to field evacuation, to a casualty collection area, to transportation to a medical facility, through the diagnostic areas, and finally to transfer to a DCA, an ongoing process called *triage* takes place. The etymology derives from the French "to sort." The decisions surrounding sorting, however, are highly situational. Initial sorting of patients attempts to identify their injury or illness and route them to appropriate care. In addition, when resources are inadequate to meet needs, triage performs a second function: rationing. Rationing is the process by which scarce resources are distributed, ideally in a prioritized manner to the most needy. Rationing is a charged topic for health care in the United States, but it is a long-recognized function of triage; however, rationing is seldom employed, because resources are rarely unavailable. Rationing decisions may occur at each of multiple points between the scene and the DCA: evacuation, first aid, transport, decontamination, admission, transfer, and treatment. If resources at each step are adequate, no rationing takes place; however, in a disaster, the closer one is to the scene when evaluating resources relative to needs, the more likely that rationing must take place.

During rapidly evolving events in the field, in transit, or on arrival to the hospital, a triage officer will attach a color-coded classification tag to each victim. Black tags designate dead or moribund victims. Victims who have serious injuries requiring immediate treatment are tagged red. Yellow tags identify patients who will eventually require treatment. Green tags signify ambulatory patients who have minor injuries. In addition, most casualties arrive from the scene untagged and with no obvious injury; however, the un-tagged patients may require decontamination and counseling. All affected victims must be observed and re-evaluated, because their condition may de-teriorate. Finally, several people arrive at the hospital untagged: media, family, bystanders, well-meaning volunteers, and, following a terrorist event, potentially people with nefarious intent.

The absolute and relative numbers of each type of victim triaged for any event will vary. The biggest variable in explosive urban events is the un-tagged mass, which depends on the number of people present, location, and time of day. Different mechanisms generate reproducible patterns of death, injury, and illness; some examples include closed-space versus open-air explosions [5] and food-borne versus airborne infectious agents. Familiarity with these patterns enables clinicians to anticipate victim type, timing, acuity, and treatment needs [6,14].

The immediate focus must be on the victims with red and yellow tags. These victims' lives hang in the balance. With timely diagnosis and appro-priate treatment in functional DCAs, most of these victims will live; without it, many will die [30].

Relevant characteristics of resources

DCA managers must assess medical resources based on whether they can or cannot maintain normal standard of care.

Resource categorization focuses on the ability to maintain standard of care and integrates with event characteristics and victim categorization. Re-sources can be categorized as normal, surge, and overflow. Normal resources define the standard of care. The authors propose a definition of surge re-sources as alternate equipment, locations, and personnel that can be used in the treatment of additional patients while maintaining the standard of care. In contrast, overflow resources are equipment, locations, and personnel that can be used in the treatment of additional patients, but which compro-mise the standard of care. As casualty loads increase, normal, surge, and overflow resources are engaged and eventually exhausted. Once all overflow resources are consumed, the system is overwhelmed. Only at this point should rationing victims' access to definitive care take place.

The surge capacity of a facility is defined simply as the total number of patients that can be managed with only normal and surge resources. Over-flow capacity is likewise defined as the absolute number of patients who can be accommodated with the addition of overflow resources. In reality, as ca-sualty loads increase during a disaster, not all resources will be exhausted while treating the same number of patients. Thus, each resource (ventilators, monitors, nursing staff, and so forth) has its own normal, surge, and over-flow capacity. For planning purposes, once a single resource of the next level must be employed, the patient should be considered as being treated within the next level's capacity. For instance, managing a critically ill patient in the postanesthesia care unit (PACU) (a surge resource) with a 1:4 nursing care ratio (overflow strategy) would be considered as using the hospital's DCA overflow capacity.

The rationale behind distinguishing these types of resources is to clarify resource management in the face of escalating needs. From this perspective, the system can be considered to be functioning continuously along a spectrum from normal to surge to overflow to overwhelmed. Many institutions use their surge capacity on a regular basis—for example, institutions that hold patients overnight in the PACU because the ICUs are full. Once surge resources are consumed, substandard practices or resources must be used to accommodate additional patients. These overflow resources are acceptable and appropriate to treat the large numbers of noncritical victims of any disaster and may be necessary even for critical victims in extreme circumstances. However, the more surge capacity (maintaining standard of care) that can be identified beforehand and quickly mobilized for critically ill and injured victims, the greater the impact will be on overall survival from the event.

Definitive care area disaster planning

The size of an event must always be placed in the context of the medical facility's normally available resources. A small event is defined as one that results in a casualty load manageable by using the involved facility's normal resources. At the opposite end of the spectrum, an extra-large event is defined as one that overwhelms the facility by generating a casualty load that cannot be accommodated even with overflow resources. The absolute numbers of casualties accommodated at each level are higher for a large urban trauma center (Table 3) than for a freestanding rural surgical center. Neither small nor extra-large events benefit from DCA planning. Small events are routinely managed with available resources, whereas extra-large events are overwhelming by definition.

A truly overwhelming mass casualty event (MCE) mandates a triage strategy that involves rationing access to definitive care. Rationing entails difficult ethical decisions. The priority becomes saving as many victims as possible given the available resources. How to render care in these austere circumstances is not in the authors' area of expertise or within the scope of this paper; but difficult decisions must be made until outside assistance arrives. Contingency planning for an overwhelming scenario does not fall on individual departments or hospitals but rather is done regionally. Rubinson and colleagues [31] published recommendations for establishing such planning to include pre-event legislative action, public transparency, and regional, rather than single hospital, implementation.

Plans developed at the DCA manager level are designed to prevent, or at least postpone, being overwhelmed. If clinicians are overwhelmed, they will

Table 3
Integration of disaster size with triage and rationing strategies

	Status			
	Normal (small event)	MCI (medium event)	MCI (large event)	MCE (extra-large event)
Resources used	Normal	Red and yellow: surge resources Green: overflow resources	Overflow resources for all	Overwhelmed situation
Rationing strategy	None	Red and yellow: no rationing Green: ration time-to-treat (acceptable to delay)	Compromise standards of care	Ration access to care
Typical numbers of victims for an urban trauma center				
Red	2	5	15	Large + 1
Yellow	4	10	30	Large + 1
Green	8	20	60+	Large + 1
Untagged	10–30	30–300	100–2000	>2000

have to do their best with what is available until outside help arrives. If care providers are overwhelmed, they should plan on providing only basic first aid and rationing access to definitive care resources [32–35].

Regarding an overwhelming event, the treatment of critically injured victims is quickly superseded in priority by public health needs, which include provisions for food, shelter, proper sanitation facilities, and clean water [36].

The focus of DCA planning efforts is on medium and large events. Medium events are those in which the critically ill or injured can be managed while maintaining standard of care with surge capacity resources. Large events can be handled only by using auxiliary substandard overflow capacity (see Table 3).

Fire, electrical failure, and flooding are internal disaster events that affect hospital infrastructure. The medical and clinical response is to maintain patient care. For the most part, plans for internal disasters are already in place; the challenges are largely administrative and logistic. The major decision during an internal disaster is whether or not to evacuate the facility [37–40]. Plans for internal disasters and evacuation must be protocol-based, formulated in advance, activated automatically, and drilled periodically [41].

Regarding external events from the perspective of the DCA, upstream triage decisions serve to screen and select from the patients who will benefit from surgery or critical care. Rationing at this level will unfortunately deny care to precisely those patients whom the triage system has selected as most likely to benefit from DCA interventions. Provision of care without rationing is the goal of DCA disaster preparedness planning.

Once the system identifies patients as critical and delivers them to a DCA, triage ceases to function as routing; ORs and ICUs are the best of what medicine has to offer. In a DCA, rationing is employed only as a last resort. It may be appropriate to offer less than optimal care to green tagged victims; they can be triaged to a cafeteria or gymnasium for observation and delayed treatment. The impact on the outcomes of these patients will be minimal, but when resources are compromised or withheld from those routed to DCAs, mortality will increase [30].

Special attention must be paid to patients already under treatment in DCAs [42]. The first impulse when a disaster strikes is to curtail surgery, and to discharge "stable" patients from ICUs. However, patients are in these areas before the disaster for good reasons. Published experience indicates that even in rapidly evolving disasters, there is adequate time (2–4 hours) [6] with a preordained plan for these areas to be prepared and expanded to accommodate the incoming surge of casualties.

Tabletop exercises

Tabletop exercises are planned rehearsals of MCIs or MCEs, organized to challenge the community and responders involved in the management of the disaster. The degree of sophistication of a tabletop exercise can range from simple to very complex. The simplest form is when a few individuals literally sit around a table and discuss the sequence of their responses to events of a hypothetical disaster based on a written scenario. More complex variations of exercises can be from the hospital [43] or regional level (which includes first responders, communication systems, and local agencies) [44,45] to national or multinational disaster rehearsals [46,47]. Common to all of these exercises are a careful pre-event plan, some degree of reality simulation, anticipation of relevant participants' responses (often a group of observers), and most importantly, a post hoc analysis of how the response was executed. Identifying the response problems and implementing the solutions are critical components of any tabletop exercise.

Tabletop exercises for DCAs are performed by appropriate administrative and clinical leadership and represent the fundamental process by which surge and overflow capacity planning occurs. The most likely disaster scenario from a hazard vulnerability analysis [48] is considered first. The process begins by identifying all the components necessary to provide care to a typical victim. Once normal resources are identified, participants identify surge and overflow resources. At each level of care (normal, surge, overflow), the care-limiting resource is identified. Participants then explore ways to expand that specific resource. The process continues by analyzing the subsequently exposed care-limiting resources. Then the exercise is repeated, assessing the next most likely scenario, and so on. When this process is completed, the group will have generated an inventory of all normal, surge, and overflow resources needed to provide each level of care in the ORs and ICUs. Within each category, a sequence of resource use is defined. For instance, the sequence of locations at Bellevue Hospital (BH) where emergency surgery can be performed (with capacity in parentheses) is as follows:

surgery normally performed in ORs (15)
surge to day surgery (2), then OB (3)
overflow to cystoscopy suites (2), angio suites (2), PACU (12), and ICU (18)

We describe the analysis of the surgical intensive care unit (SICU) capacity at BH to illustrate the process. BH recently opened a new 10-bed SICU and an 8-bed step-down unit. In 2001, during the design phase, the team decided to build the 8 step-down rooms identical to, interchangeable with, and adjacent to the 10 SICU rooms. Consequently, we can now immediately increase our ICU capacity from 10 to 18 beds by simply providing additional staffing. We consider these 18 beds our initial ICU surge capacity, achieved through the dual usage of our step-down beds. Once those 18 beds are full, the resources listed in Table 4 are necessary to provide critical care, with the additional surge capacity alternatives:

We would use anesthesia machines for ventilators. Wall oxygen would be augmented with oxygen tanks. Additional ICU beds could be located in other ICUs the PACU and ORs, and we have cooperative transfer agreements with neighboring and affiliated hospitals. Housestaff would be reassigned from ambulatory and elective rotations. Nursing administration would provide overtime, use agencies, and tap float pools to maintain staffing. With these measures, nurse staffing is our surge capacity-limiting resource. In fact, this is often our normal capacity-limiting resource. We have the physical capacity, equipment, and medical staff to care simultaneously for 96 critically ill patients with up to two thirds of these patients ventilated. Our nursing department estimates capacity to care for only a maximum of about 50 patients with a 2:1 ICU staffing ratio. Consequently, our surge capacity expansion efforts have endeavored to increase nurse staffing.

Table 4
ICU surge capacity

Resource	Standard of care alternatives
Ventilators	Anesthesia machines, regional resources in 48 h
Wall O_2	O_2 tanks
ICU beds	Other ICUs, PACU, ORs, transfers
House staff	Reassign
Nursing staff[a]	Overtime, agency, float

[a] Capacity-limiting resource.

We enter the overflow capacity phase (substandard alternatives) for each of these resources as they are consumed. Table 5 describes our response for each resource.

Bag-valve-mask resuscitators would substitute for ventilators; supplemental oxygen would be abandoned for room air; and patients would be located wherever there was space. Housestaff work hour regulations would be violated and the nurse/staffing ratio exceeded. In our overflow capacity scenario, it is the number of actual beds that limits our capacity. Using these resources, we estimate being able to care for about 200 critical patients for at most 48 hours, at which time outside relief would be required. This assistance would be expected from either regional cooperative arrangements or from Strategic National Stockpile resources.

It is important to involve all clinical services and areas in these exercises to anticipate problems where surge resources overlap. An anesthesia machine in a cystoscopy suite cannot serve to expand ICU ventilator capacity at the same time that surgeons are planning on using that room to expand trauma surgical capacity.

In addition, it is imperative that all clinical support services (radiology, blood bank, laboratory services, pharmacy, dietary, sterile supply, and so forth) collaborate in these iterative tabletop exercises. During the 2003 electrical blackout at BH, we discovered that our sterile equipment processing was not on the emergency backup generator, and BH no longer supports gas sterilization. Because the blackout began at 4 PM on a Thursday, most surgical instruments were either in use or dirty. Consequently, capacity to perform multiple operations was severely curtailed; fortunately, only two patients required emergency operations during the blackout.

The process of continuously identifying the capacity- or care-limiting resource is crucial. Expansion planning can then focus on that weak link. It makes no sense to devote time and energy to expanding one resource, like ORs, when their usage will be limited by lack of sterile instruments.

The advantage of defining relevant aspects of events, victims, and resources as described, and of adopting the tabletop system for developing resource expansion, is that the resulting plans can be considered to be in daily use. It is likely that several times per year, surge and even overflow resources may be needed simply due to the normal variations in admissions and

Table 5
ICU overflow capacity

Resource	Suboptimal alternatives
Ventilators	Hand ventilate with bag-valve-mask device
Wall O$_2$	Room air
ICU beds[a]	General wards, hallways
House staff	Work hour regulation noncompliance
Nursing staff	1:3+ staffing ratio, non-ICU nurses

[a] Capacity-limiting resource.

acuity. Incorporating disaster preparedness vernacular and algorithms into daily clinical usage maintains preparedness at a continuously high level.

A number of concepts regarding the medical DCA response to disaster have been presented. The goals are threefold. The first goal is to define an understandable vocabulary and to create a usable framework to simplify and focus planning of the tasks at hand. The second goal is to provide tools and strategies to use in developing plans for a clinical response to disaster. The final goal is to present some of the remaining challenges that seriously threaten the ability to care for patients in DCAs, and which have major consequences on overall mortality following any given event. By exposing these challenges, we hope to inspire DCA clinicians to become involved in departmental, hospital, and regional planning.

Acknowledgment

The authors wish to thank Meghan E. Sise and Erick J. Arbenz, MD, for their contributions to this manuscript.

References

[1] Hirshberg A, Holcomb JB, Mattox KL. Hospital trauma care in multiple-casualty incidents: a critical view. Ann Emerg Med 2001;37:647–52.
[2] Cushman JG, Pachter L, Beaton HL. Two New York City hospitals' surgical response to the September 11, 2001, terrorist attack in New York City. J Trauma 2003;54:147–55.
[3] Feeney JM, Goldberg R, Blumenthal JA, et al. September 11, 2001, revisited. Arch Surg 2005;140:1068–73.
[4] Marcus SG, Shamamian P, Cushman J. Remembering September 11: reflections from Bellevue Hospital and New York University Medical Center. Surgery 2002;132(3):502–5.
[5] Kluger Y, Peleg K, Daniel-Aharonson L, et al. Israeli Trauma Group. The special injury pattern in terrorist bombings. J Am Coll Surg 2004;199:875–9.
[6] Shamir MY, Weiss YG, Willner D, et al. Multiple casualty terror events: the anesthesiologist's perspective. Anesth Analg 2004;98:1746–52.
[7] Frykberg ER. Medical management of disasters and mass casualties from terrorist bombings: how can we cope? J Trauma 2002;53:201–12.
[8] Gutierrez de Ceballos JP, Turegano Fuentes F, Perez Diaz D, et al. Casualties treated at the closest hospital in the Madrid, March 11, terrorist bombings. Crit Care Med 2005;33: S107–12.
[9] Holden PJP. Improvising in an emergency. N Engl J Med 2005;353(6):541–3.
[10] Ryan J, Montgomery H. Terrorism and the medical response. N Engl J Med 2005;353(6): 543–5.
[11] Magee M, editor. All available boats. The evacuation of Manhattan Island on September 11, 2001. New York: Spencer Books; 2002.
[12] Frykberg ER, Tepas JJ III. Terrorist bombings: lessons learned from Belfast to Beirut. Ann Surg 1988;208:569–76.
[13] O'Toole T. Congress of the United States and U.S. Senate Government Affairs Subcommittee on International Security, Proliferation and Federal Services Hearing on FEMA's Role in Managing Bioterrorist Attacks and the Impact of Public Health Concerns on Bioterrorism Preparedness testimony. July 23, 2001. Available at: http://www.upmc-biosecurity.org/pages/resources/hearings/otoole_02.html. Accessed April 17, 2006.

[14] Roccaforte JD, Cushman JG. Disaster preparation and management for the intensive care unit. Curr Opin Crit Care 2002;8:607–15.

[15] Kamarck E. Testimony to the Judiciary Committee of the United States Senate. November 14, 2002. Available at: http://www.ksg.harvard.edu/news/onthehill/2002/kamarck_111402.htm. Accessed April 17, 2006.

[16] Smithson AE, Levy LA. Ataxia: The chemical and biological terrorism threat and the U.S. response. The Henry L. Stimson Center Report No. 35, October 2000. Available at: http://www.stimson.org/pubs.cfm?ID=12. Accessed April 17, 2006.

[17] Barbera JA, Macintyre AG, DeAtley CA. Ambulances to nowhere: America's critical short-fall in medical preparedness for catastrophic terrorism. BCSIA Discussion Paper 2001-15, ESDP Discussion Paper ESDP-2001-07, John F. Kennedy School of Government, Harvard University, October 2001. Available at: http://www.gwu.edu/~icdrm/publications/index.html. Accessed April 17, 2006.

[18] Hogan C. Responding to a fire at a pediatric hospital. AORN J 2002;75(4):793–800.

[19] Prezant DJ, Clair J, Belyaev S, et al. Effects of the August 2003 blackout on the New York City healthcare delivery system: a lesson for disaster preparedness. Crit Care Med 2005;33(1 Suppl):S96–101.

[20] Klein KR, Rosenthal MS, Klausner HA. Blackout 2003: preparedness and lessons learned from the perspectives of four hospitals. Prehospital Disaster Med 2005;20(5):343–9.

[21] Berggren RE, Curiel TJ. After the storm—health care infrastructure in post-Katrina New Orleans. N Engl J Med 2006;354(15):1549–52.

[22] Cocanour CS, Allen SJ, Mazabob J, et al. Lessons learned from the evacuation of an urban teaching hospital. Arch Surg 2002;137(10):1141–5.

[23] Arnold JL, Halpern P, Tsai MC, et al. Mass casualty terrorist bombings: a comparison of outcomes by bombing type. Ann Emerg Med 2004;43(2):263–73.

[24] Almogy G, Belzberg H, Mintz Y, et al. Suicide bombing attacks: update and modifications to the protocol. Ann Surg 2004;239(3):295–303.

[25] Emami MJ, Tavakoli AR, Alemzadeh H, et al. Strategies in evaluation and management of Bam earthquake victims. Prehospital Disaster Med 2005;20(5):327–30.

[26] Hawryluck L, Lapinsky SE, Stewart TE. Clinical review: SARS—lessons in disaster management. Crit Care 2005;9(4):384–9.

[27] U.S. National Weather Service. National Hurricane Center, Katrina Advisory Archive. August 23–29, 2005. Available at: http://www.nhc.noaa.gov/archive/2005/KATRINA.shtml. Accessed April 17, 2006.

[28] World Health Organization, Disease Outbreak News. Update 83—one hundred days into the outbreak, June 18, 2003. Available at: http://www.who.int/csr/don/2003_06_18/en/index.html. Accessed April 17, 2006.

[29] Committee on Trauma. Resources for optimal care of the injured patient. Chicago: American College of Surgeons; 1993.

[30] Simchen E, Sprung CL, Galai N, et al. Survival of critically ill patients hospitalized in and out of intensive care units under paucity of intensive care unit beds. Crit Care Med 2004;32:1654–61.

[31] Rubinson L, Nuzzo JB, Talmor DS, et al. Augmentation of hospital critical care capacity after bioterrorist attacks or epidemics: recommendations of the Working Group on Emergency Mass Critical Care. Crit Care Med 2005;33(10):2393–403.

[32] Hick JL, Hanfling D, Burstein JL, et al. Health care facility and community strategies for patient care surge capacity. Ann Emerg Med 2004;44(3):253–61.

[33] Agency for Healthcare Research and Quality. Prepared by Health Systems Research Inc. under Contract No. 290-04-0010. Altered standards of care in mass casualty events. AHRQ Publication 05-0043. Rockville (MD); 2005.

[34] Hick JL, O'Laughlin DT. Concept of operations for triage of mechanical ventilation in an epidemic. Acad Emerg Med 2006;13(2):223–9.

[35] Koenig KL, Cone DC, Burstein JL, et al. Surging to the right standard of care. Acad Emerg Med 2006;13(2):195–8.

[36] Brodie M, Weltzien E, Altman D, et al. Experiences of Hurricane Katrina evacuees in Houston shelters: implications for future planning. Am J Public Health 2006;96(8):1402–8.

[37] Sternberg E, Lee GC, Huard D. Counting crises: US hospital evacuations, 1971-1999. Prehospital Disaster Med 2004;19(2):150–7.

[38] Schultz CH, Koenig KL, Lewis RJ. Implications of hospital evacuation after the Northridge, California earthquake. N Engl J Med 2003;348:1349–55.

[39] Berman MA, Lazar EJ. Hospital emergency preparedness—lessons learned since Northridge. N Engl J Med 2003;348:1307–8.

[40] Augustine J, Schoettmer JT. Evacuation of a rural community hospital: lessons learned from an unplanned event. Disaster Manag Response 2005;3(3):68–72.

[41] Klein JS, Weigelt JA. Disaster management, lessons learned. Surg Clin North Am 1991;71: 257–66.

[42] Sinuff T, Kahnamoui K, Cook DJ, et al. Values ethics and rationing in critical care task force. Rationing critical care beds: a systematic review. Crit Care Med 2004;32:1588–97.

[43] Cosgrove SE, Jenckes MW, Kohri D, et al. Evaluation of hospital disaster drills: a module-based approach. Prepared by Johns Hopkins University Evidence-Based Practice Center under Contract No. 290-02-0018. AHRQ Publication No. 04-0032. Agency for Healthcare Research and Quality. Rockville (MD); 2004.

[44] Taylor JL, Roup BJ, Blythe D, et al. Pandemic influenza preparedness in Maryland: improving readiness through a tabletop exercise. Biosecur Bioterror 2005;3(1):61–9.

[45] Jasper E, Miller M, Sweeney B, et al. Preparedness of hospitals to respond to a radiological terrorism event as assessed by a full-scale exercise. J Public Health Manag Pract 2005;(Suppl): S11–6.

[46] Smith BT, Inglesby TV, Brimmer E, et al. Navigating the storm: report and recommendations from the Atlantic Storm exercise. Biosecur Bioterror 2005;3(3):256–67.

[47] Jacobs LM, Burns KJ. Terrorism preparedness: web-based resource management and the TOPOFF 3 exercise. J Trauma 2006;60(3):566–71.

[48] Joint Commission on Accreditation of Healthcare Organizations. Special issue, emergency management in the new millenium. Jt Comm Perspect 2001;21(12):8–9. Available at: http://wwwjcrinc.com/perspectivesspecialissue. Accessed April 17, 2006.

ELSEVIER
SAUNDERS

Anesthesiology Clin
25 (2007) 179–188

ANESTHESIOLOGY
CLINICS

Multiple Casualty Incidents: The Prehospital Role of the Anesthesiologist in Europe

David J. Baker, DM, FRCA*, Caroline Telion, MD
Pierre Carli, MD, PhD

*Department of Anesthesiology and SAMU de Paris, Hôpital Necker – Enfants Malades,
149 rue de Sèvres, 75743 Paris CEDEX 15, France*

During the past 50 years, mass casualty incidents in civil life have occurred regularly, both as a result of accidents and, more recently, from terrorist activity. The management of mass casualties is of continuing concern [1]. Urban terrorism is a problem faced by a number of countries around the world, including those in Europe [2–6]. Trauma surgery and anesthesia have been developed to treat casualties from such incidents after they have reached hospital. Emergency response plans have also been developed universally to provide a coordinated prehospital emergency response. Differences in these plans in Europe reflect different approaches to the provision of emergency medical care. Anesthesiologists have been involved increasingly in primary management, particularly in France where they have been an integral part of the emergency medical service Service d'Aide Medicale Urgente (SAMU) for more than 30 years [7]. Lessons learned from military anesthesia and emergency hospital management have been brought forward in the chain of care by anesthesiologists whose training has a wide academic base and particular skills that are important in the immediate management of mass casualties.

Increasingly, during the past 30 years, regular terrorist attacks involving improvised explosive devices have occurred that have caused mass casualties from blast and penetrating injury. The terrorist bombings in London in 2005 and in Paris in 1995 highlighted the special problems facing the emergency services working in a confined space [2–4]. The explosions caused by suicide bus and car bombers in Israel and Iraq in recent years, which have

---

* Corresponding author.
  E-mail address: 113445.3600@wanadoo.fr (D.J. Baker).

doi:10.1016/j.atc.2006.11.006

lead to widespread injury and loss of life, have been in the open. In contrast, underground explosions lead to a magnification of blast, burns, and inhalational injury, and cause very difficult and dangerous conditions of access and rescue for emergency responders. As a consequence, the dangers of blast injury and secondary chemical hazards are receiving renewed focus [8].

The pattern of trauma in civil practice depends on geographic location. In certain countries, such as the United States, penetrating trauma is relatively common because of the violent nature of urban life in some areas. In Europe, until recently, blunt trauma has been more prevalent. The relevance for mass casualty management is in the lessons provided by individual blunt and penetrating trauma management in prehospital and hospital management, which can be translated into mass casualty management.

This article considers the management of mass casualties in terms of planning and delivery of care, and the specific prehospital role of the anesthesiologist in trauma management, based on experiences in Europe.

Mechanisms of injury

Mass casualty incidents involve numerous mechanisms of injury, including penetrating and blunt trauma. Penetration may be caused by stab wounds and low- and high-velocity bullets, each presenting with their own clinical signatures. Blunt injury is caused predominately by motor vehicle accidents. Accidental and deliberate explosions cause both blunt and penetrating injury as part of the four stages of blast [8]. In this situation, trauma may be complicated by burning, both external and in the respiratory tract. Chemical injury (which may be regarded as toxic trauma [9]) occurs most often from self-poisoning, but mass casualties are usually the result of accidental or deliberate chemical release. Many somatic systems are affected by chemical exposure, with the respiratory and nervous systems producing life-threatening effects [10]. In addition to physical and chemical trauma, damage may be the result of exposure to ionizing radiation from accidental or deliberate release using an improvised explosive device.

Areas of concern to the anesthesiologist

In both physical and toxic trauma, damage to critical anatomic sites and somatic systems (ie, the chest, lungs, and head) may mean an immediate threat to life. In physical trauma, the cardiorespiratory system is a critical target. Other sites, such as the abdomen, limbs, and peripheral nerves, pose a relative risk in terms of physical trauma, although the nervous system is a critical site for certain chemical agents. The anesthesiologist, because of his/her training and experience, is well-adapted to the early management of all these forms of trauma, particularly in providing life-support stabilization for physical trauma, and his/her understanding of the detailed physiology and pharmacology of the respiratory, cardiac, and nervous systems.

The anesthesiologist is concerned with the management of several pathophysiologic mechanisms in toxic and traumatic trauma. Shock, with tissue hypoxia and lactic acidosis, is common in blunt and penetrating injury, but tissue hypoxia is also the final common pathway of toxic trauma [10]. Lung edema may be the result of direct blast injury [8] or exposure to chemical agents. Early activation of the kinin cascade in lung injury may provoke later onset of respiratory complications such as acute respiratory distress syndrome [11]. Factors determining on-site management of mass casualties include accessibility and entrapment, conscious level, airway and ventilation, pain, and circulatory damage. Responding to mass casualties from deliberate causes also involves dangers to the responders from potential sequelae of the primary cause, such as a second terrorist explosive device targeting the responders, and persistent, transmissible chemical hazards.

Planning for mass casualties

Essential stages are required for the initial treatment of both limited numbers and mass casualties, which are incorporated into management systems such as advanced life support and advanced trauma life support. The latter system, widely taught and used in the United States, has proved popular in the United Kingdom and other English-speaking countries, but is not used in many other European countries, notably France. There, anesthesiologists are involved closely in the application of advanced trauma life support measures, including airway, ventilation, and definitive circulatory access. As elsewhere in the world, the objectives are the prevention of further injury and starting immediate life-saving measures. In addition, the patient is prepared for safe onward transport to emergency hospital facilities with physical stabilization for multiple trauma. In France, general anesthesia or intravenous analgesia and sedation usually are given on-site for victims with multiple trauma and head injury (see later discussion).

Approaches to prehospital organization in Europe

In Europe, as in other parts of the world, prehospital care is divided between systems that are paramedically and medically operated. In the United Kingdom, ambulance services are based essentially on paramedics, although physicians, including anesthesiologists, are sent from hospitals in mass casualty incidents and as part of a few helicopter services operating in London [3] and other parts of the country. However, the ambulance services in the United Kingdom are not organized on a national basis, nor are they part of the hospital service. Although each regional service has its own medical director, links with other doctors, including anesthesiologists, are not formalized. Many hospital specialists have, however, built good links with the ambulance services and a voluntary organization British Association for Immediate Care (BASICS) allows physicians to help ambulance services on-site at major incidents on a voluntary basis. The fact that emergency services are not operated on a nationally controlled basis means that there are no national emergency plans comparable with those in France. Instead, each hospital governing organization is responsible for producing its own plan.

The tube and bus attacks in London in July 2005 resulted in a realization of the value of an on-site medical presence for major incidents. The helicopter emergency medical service was dispatched using a helicopter and fast cars to several incident sites in central London [3]. At the time of writing, there is momentum toward increasing the medical presence at mass casualty incidents, both for physical injury and for the victims of chemical agent release. In the July incidents, anesthesiologists provided on-site general anesthesia for entrapped casualties in the deep tube (underground railway) system.

Anesthesiologists and the emergency medical services response: the French approach

In France, anesthesiologists are an integral part of the emergency medical system (SAMU), which was founded in 1970 by Professor Louis Lareng in Toulouse [7]. The idea behind SAMU is to have a service manned by physicians, both in dispatching and in on-site provision of care. SAMU aims to bring the hospital to the patient. This process is aided by the fact that many SAMU units operate from hospitals and that the medical staff involved in running them are also employed within hospital services. Prehospital disaster care in France is controlled by two national response plans, "the red plan" [12] and "the white plan" [13,14]. The red plan concerns the rescue and evacuation of victims from a disaster site by the fire and rescue service. The plan provides for an overall on-site commander who controls a fire and rescue and a medical chain. The commander reports to the prefect of the department (in Paris, to the prefect of police) who then reports directly to the prime minister. The fire and rescue chain, under the control of the director of fire and rescue, is concerned with managing the cause of the disaster, rescuing victims and providing essential primary medical care using their own internal medical resources (all French fire services have medical units and firefighters are trained to emergency medical technician levels). Firefighters rescue victims in a shuttle operation (*le petit noria* or "small waterwheel") and deliver them to the medical chain at the advanced medical post distant from the site of the disaster. The AMP is under the overall control of the director of medical rescue, who is usually a fire service medical officer (these are a feature of the French system). Running of the AMP is the responsibility of a physician chosen by the director of medical rescue, whose responsibilities include triage, immediate casualty care, and secondary evacuation of the patients to designated hospitals (*le grand noria* or "big waterwheel") (Fig. 1).

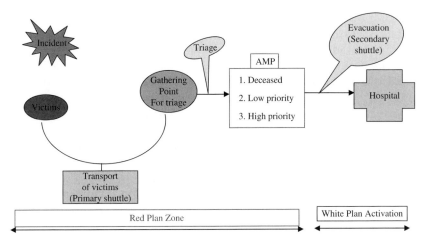

Fig. 1. Interaction of the red and white plans in France for the evacuation of casualties after a disaster.

At this point, the white plan [13,14] begins. This plan is concerned essentially with hospital response to mass casualties caused by disaster. Its provisions include setting up crisis management cells, recalling personnel, freeing hospital resources, and organizing controlled reception of mass casualties. The organization of French emergency medical services allows a particular approach to incidents involving mass casualties. The ambulance services (SAMU) are controlled and manned medically, which allows a number of on-site emergency measures not provided easily by services led by paramedic staff. Thus, patients receive a great degree of care before arriving at the hospital. In addition, the SAMU and hospital services are operated by the same organization (in Paris, this is the Assistance Publique–Hopitaux de Paris), which allows integration of planning and a continuum of care from the prehospital to the hospital under the control of hospital doctors who also control the SAMU.

The integration of prehospital and hospital services provided by the white plan means that the hospital can effectively be extended beyond its boundaries by sending the SAMU mobile medical units to the scene of the disaster where they link up with the fire service operating the red plan. In effect, therefore, the AMP is the interface between the on-site and hospital management of casualties.

Special planning for chemical releases

After the toxic attack in Japan in 1995, many countries around the world considered planning options in case further terrorist attacks should take place. In France, detailed planning (Plan Piratox) had been put in place in 1987 as a special modification of the red plan to deal with chemical releases. Plan Piratox provides for detection, triage, and decontamination of casualties by fire fighters in a contaminated zone, while providing essential first aid. Decontaminated casualties are then delivered to the SAMU at the AMP in the non-contaminated zone. The plan was revised in further government circulars issued in 2002 [15], with special reference to the management of possible terrorist chemical, biological, radiologic, and nuclear (CBRN) incidents. At the same time, another circular [16] was issued to provide specific instructions to hospitals for the management of mass casualties from CBRN incidents (Plan Biotox). This circular was, in effect, an updating of the white plan. These circulars contain not only organizational flowcharts, but also technical annexes that contain definitive medical and scientific data about the management of patients exposed to the main toxic hazards.

In the government circulars of 2002, the role of special receiving hospitals is clearly defined. France is divided administratively into seven "defense zones." For each of these, organization for response to CBRN incidents is under the direct control of the defense zone administrator (Prefect). In each zone, key hospitals (termed "reference hospitals") are designated to take chemical–biological casualties. They are chosen because they contain, as part of their normal daily work, expertise and facilities that can be used quickly in the event of a CBRN incidents. These establishments are essentially the head of an extensive referral system that includes the SAMU ambulance services and its constituent stations; the SAMU of each region is coordinated by the reference hospital. In addition, the reference hospital is linked to specialist poisons centers, infectious disease facilities, nuclear medical facilities, and occupational health organizations to provide a broad spectrum approach to CBRN releases.

Prehospital anesthesia for mass casualty incidents

Analgesia is administered frequently at the site of the emergency, and early analgesia should be a priority for trauma cases. In the SAMU system, analgesics used include morphine itself and mixed opioid agonist/antagonist drugs such as nalbuphine, together with nonopioid compounds. Regional anesthesia is used, and crural or brachial plexus block with lidocaine is administered routinely by trained anesthesiologists in the case of fractures of the extremities. General anesthesia has many advantages in the management of major trauma. Indications include extrication of a trapped patient, intractable restlessness, and severe head trauma with presumed elevated intracranial pressure. All trauma patients should be assumed to have a full stomach, and a rapid sequence induction is used routinely with succinylcholine. In trauma cases, cricoid pressure with manual in-line stabilization is used only after the anesthetist has considered the possibility of risking further cervical spine injury against that of aspiration pneumonia. General anesthesia requires drugs suitable for a hypotensive trauma patient, and ketamine, etomidate, and low doses of midazolam are the most commonly used.

Continuing care by Service d'Aide Medicale Urgente

After carrying out the essential measures required for stabilization of the emergency, the medical ICU (MICU) physician transmits a detailed appraisal of the patient to the medical regulator by radio. The patient is then transported to the designated hospital that has the service best suited to the case. In some cities, serious cases of trauma are sent to a special trauma center, where its trauma team, accurately briefed by the SAMU medical dispatcher, is ready to receive them. Should the patient's condition deteriorate suddenly during ground transportation, the vehicle is halted temporarily while the patient is destabilized.

The time spent on-site by the MICU depends very much on the nature of the emergency. Cases of blunt trauma are stabilized for airway, ventilation, and circulatory support before transport to hospital, but cases of penetrating trauma are transported quickly to a suitable surgical service, after quickly securing the airway and ventilation and establishing intravenous access. Like the dispatching system of SAMU, the nature of the on-site response is also highly flexible and depends on standard clinical decisions made by the doctor in the MICU.

Controversies in prehospital care

Prehospital emergency management, particularly of trauma, remains a particularly controversial issue and is the subject of much discussion and debate. Essentially, the United State prehospital care system, which is based on the use of paramedics, is based on the theory of rapid evacuation of the patient to a specialized center (the so-called "scoop and run" approach), whereas in some European systems, on-site stabilization is predominant. Although medical conditions such as coronary syndromes and cardiac arrest show a clear benefit from immediate on-site treatment by such techniques as fibrinolysis and defibrillation, analysis of the different approaches to trauma patients is more difficult, particularly in comparing the practices in the United States and Europe.

The first point for consideration in the analysis is the prevalence of the type of trauma encountered. Penetrating trauma from knife and gunshot wounds is far more common in the United States than in Europe, where blunt trauma predominates. In shocked open trauma patients, many trauma surgeons in the United States consider intravenous fluid therapy in the prehospital setting to be ineffective, time consuming, and possibly deleterious. This view has received support from a large-scale, randomized study [17], which included only hypotensive patients suffering from penetrating truncal injury and which appeared to demonstrate the adverse effect on outcome and recovery of prehospital volume loading. The patients who did not receive prehospital intravenous fluid therapy apparently had a significantly better outcome (70% versus 62% survival). However, the results do not clearly state the causes of death, and the selection of patients may have been biased.

Controversy also exists regarding the time required by a paramedic to start an IV line, and the efficacy of IV line placement, which are dependent on skills and experience. However, the optimal blood pressure for a patient bleeding from uncontrolled hemorrhage is still a matter of debate [18]. Many trauma surgeons argue that a patient who has a low perfusion pressure from hypovolemia is liable to less subsequent hemorrhage than if the blood pressure is raised using volume expanders.

The stabilization of respiratory distress on-scene, however, is less controversial. Efficient respiratory management has been shown to be a major advantage of prehospital stabilization, whether in rapid evacuation or in on-site stabilization.

Endotracheal intubation and tension pneumothorax decompression on-scene has been shown to reduce the incidence of early deaths in trauma [19]. In French studies, the rate of success of oral intubation by French pre-hospital medical teams has been shown to approach that attained in the operating theater, with less than a 1.4% failure. Initial management of a patient who has severe closed head trauma also requires aggressive volume resuscitation or vasoactive drugs to maintain the cerebral perfusion pressure, which is related directly to the mean arterial blood pressure [20]. Severe brain trauma modifies the hemodynamic response to hypotension because there is a failure in the cerebrovascular autoregulation. It is well known that hypoxia and hypotension following severe brain trauma worsens the prognosis.

These clinical examples show that in the SAMU system, the time used at the site to stabilize the patient is not lost. Rather, it decreases the duration of treatment after arrival in the emergency room of the hospital, and allows direct transport to specialized services where necessary [21].

Recent mass casualty incidents in Europe involving anesthesiologists: lessons learned

The Paris bombings in 1995 were managed by the combination of the red and white emergency plans and confirmed the value of having such plans in place before incidents occur. Casualties in the Paris underground bombings were managed by on-site SAMU emergency medical physicians operating from mobile ICUs according to standard SAMU practice, allowing on-site stabilization and the provision of general anesthesia and emergency surgery where necessary.

Lessons to be learned from the recent London bombings and the 1995 attacks are

- The importance of the provision of on-site emergency medical personnel who can triage patients and provide early definitive life support and

general anesthesia for polytrauma, allowing rapid extrication and transfer to early surgical support
- The importance of being able to provide emergency medical services care as close as possible to the scene of injury. The Paris bombings were similar in their nature to the Metropolitan Line bombings in London because these are both cut and cover subway systems with wide tunnels and relatively good access compared with the tube railway. The ability to set up an advanced medical post close to the incident has also been confirmed
- The importance of having integrated emergency response plans for the fire and emergency medical services

Summary

The increase in incidents involving mass casualties in recent years from accidental and terrorist causes has emphasized the need for a planned and coordinated prehospital emergency medical response.

Emergency medical care is approached in different ways in Europe, but recent terrorist attacks have emphasized the value of having medical teams on-site to provide advanced trauma life support. Although controversies still exist about the provision of prehospital emergency care, early airway and ventilation management has been shown to be of vital importance. Anesthesiologists' skills are particularly appropriate here, along with vascular access and the provision of on-site general anesthesia and analgesia.

The United Kingdom's emergency medical services system is paramedically based, like that in the United States, and bases its management on rapid evacuation of casualties to hospital emergency medical facilities. However, the London bombings in July 2005 showed the value of on-site medical teams that included anesthesiologists.

In contrast, the French emergency medical service is controlled and operated medically, and on-site provision of teams containing anesthesiologists is routine. In mass casualty incidents, these teams can work effectively with rescue personnel through the operation of national emergency response plans (red and white), which have been updated recently to respond to the continuing terrorist threat and to the threat of the release of chemical and biological agents.

References

[1] Burkle FM. Mass casualty management of large scale bioterrorist events: an epidemiological approach that shapes triage decisions. Emerg Med Clin North Am 2002;20:409–36.
[2] Carli P, Telion C, Baker D. Terrorism in France. Prehospital Disaster Med 2003;18:92–9.
[3] Lockey DJ, MacKenzie R, Redhead J, et al. London bombings July 2005: the immediate pre- hospital medical response. Resuscitation 2005;66:ix–xii.
[4] Ryan J, Montgomery H. The London attacks and preparedness: terrorism and the medical response. N Engl J Med 2005;353(6):543–5.

[5] Singer P, Cohen JD, Stein M. Conventional terrorism and critical care. Crit Care Med 2005; 33(Suppl):S61–6.

[6] de Ceballos JP, Turegano-Fuentes F, Perez-Diaz D, et al. 11 March 2004: the terrorist bomb explosions in Madrid, Spain—an analysis of the logistics, injuries sustained and clinical management of casualties treated at the closest hospital. Crit Care 2005;9(1):104–11.

[7] Carli PA, Riou B, Barriot P. Trauma anesthesia practices throughout the world: France. In: Grande CM, editor. Textbook of trauma anesthesia and critical care. St. Louis (MO): Mosby–Year Book Inc.; 1993. p.199–204 [Chapter 17].

[8] De Palma RG, Burris DG, Champion HR, et al. Blast injury. N Engl J Med 2005;352: 1335–42.

[9] Baker DJ. Chemical and biological warfare agents: the role of the anesthesiologist. In: Miller RD, editor. Anesthesia. New York: Churchill Livingstone; 2005 p. 2497–525 [Chapter 62].

[10] Baker DJ. Aspects of critical care following toxic agent release. Crit Care Med 2005; 33(Suppl):S66–74.

[11] Lachman B. The concept of open lung management. International Journal of Intensive Care 2000;7(4):215–20.

[12] Plan Rouge: an introduction. Available at: http://en.wikipedia.org/wiki/Plan_rouge [in English]. Accessed May 2006.

[13] Plan Blanc. Available at: http://www.sante.gouv.fr/htm/actu/31_030814b.htm [in French]. Accessed May 2006.

[14] Plan Blanc: an introduction. Available at: http://en.wikipedia.org/wiki/Plan_blanc [in English]. Accessed May 2006.

[15] Circulaire DHOS/HFD No 2002/284 de 3 mai 2002 relative à l'organisation du systeme hospitalier en cas d'afflux de victims. Available at: http://www.sante.gouv.fr/htm/pointsur/attentat/circ_020503.pdf [in French]. Accessed May 2006.

[16] Plan Biotox 5th October 2001: an introduction. Available at: http://www.sante.gouv.fr/htm/dossiers/biotox.intro.htm [in French]. Accessed May 2006.

[17] Bickell W, Wall M, Pepe P, et al. Immediate versus delayed fluid resuscitation for hypotensive patients with penetrating torso injuries. N Engl J Med 1994;331:1105–9.

[18] Kowalenko T, Stern S, Dronen S, et al. Improved outcome with hypotensive resuscitation of uncontrolled hemorrhagic shock in a swine model. J Trauma 1992;33:349–53.

[19] Schmidt U, Frame S, Nerlich M, et al. On-scene helicopter transport of patients with multiple injuries—comparison of a German and an American system. J Trauma 1992;33:548–55.

[20] Chesnut R, Marshall L, Klauber M, et al. The role of secondary brain injury in determining outcome from severe head injury. J Trauma 1993;34:216–20.

[21] Yates D, Carli P, Woodford M, et al. [Towards comparison of French and British system of initial trauma care]. Journal européen des urgences 1994;2:88–93 [in French].

ANESTHESIOLOGY
CLINICS

ELSEVIER
SAUNDERS

Anesthesiology Clin
25 (2007) 189–199

Nonconventional Terror—The Anesthesiologist's Role in a Nerve Agent Event

Daniel Talmor, MD, MPH

*Department of Anesthesia and Critical Care, Beth Israel Deaconess Medical Center,
Harvard Medical School, 1 Deaconess Road, CC-470, Boston, MA 02215, USA*

Overview of chemical agents

Chemical compounds capable of producing injury and death in humans are widely available. From the perspective of the clinician, there may be little difference between a terrorist event and an industrial accident. Both may involve large numbers of casualties, up to the thousands, depending on the method of agent dispersal. Both may involve dispersal by an explosion, thus producing conventionally injured patients as well as those with mixed chemical and conventional injuries. In both scenarios the strain placed on the hospital and the clinicians involved will be enormous. The skills available to the anesthesiologist in airway management and resuscitation will make anesthesia providers a critical resource in the health care system response to such an event. Prior knowledge and understanding of the agents involved, the pathophysiology of the injuries incurred, and the methods of treatment of these injuries will allow early recognition and treatment of the victims [1].

Classification of chemical agents

Chemical agents are designated as lethal or nonlethal agents. The lethal agents are designed to produce injury or death, whereas the nonlethal agents incapacitate the victim but do not usually cause death. Lethal agents are traditionally divided into four categories: nerve agents or anticholinesterases, vesicants or blistering agents, choking or pulmonary agents, and cyanogens or "blood" agents. It is important to realize that although this classification is correct for the military agents, it is not necessarily all encompassing when

---

E-mail address: dtalmor@bidmc.harvard.edu

1932-2275/07/$ - see front matter © 2007 Elsevier Inc. All rights reserved.
doi:10.1016/j.anclin.2006.12.004 *anesthesiology.theclinics.com*

dealing with agents that may be encountered in an industrial accident. However, the effects from industrial agents will generally parallel those from military agents.

Identification of a specific chemical agent

The arrival of multiple patients acutely suffering from a similar symptom complex should raise the suspicion of a chemical mass casualty event. Such an event may or may not be accompanied by an explosion. A high index of suspicion is needed and rapid action must be taken not only to treat the casualties but also to protect the health care facility and simultaneously allow time to organize an effective response.

Decontamination and supportive care will be needed for patients who have had any chemical exposure; however only nerve agents and cyanogens have specific antidotes that must be administered rapidly. Failure to immediately recognize the disease complex and to administer the appropriate medications will significantly increase both morbidity and mortality. These agents, fortunately, have specific clinical symptom complexes, which allow such a rapid clinical diagnosis and do not require complicated testing.

Nerve agents

The nerve agents include GA (tabun), GB (sarin), GD (soman), GF, and VX. These agents were first synthesized in Germany before the Second World War, hence their classification as German agent A and so on. VX was developed in the United Kingdom following the war. During the cold war, massive quantities of nerve agents were produced in both the former Soviet Union as well as in the western countries.

As weapons of war, the only known use of nerve agents was during the Iran–Iraq conflict and the subsequent suppression of ethnic minorities in Iraq. Reliable clinical data on the medical consequences of these attacks are lacking. The single dispersal of nerve agents in a country that had modern medical care was during the attack on the Tokyo subway using sarin in 1995. Although valuable lessons for the medical system may be learned from this attack, the agent used was dilute, and the resultant number of fatalities in relation to the number exposed was small. This makes it difficult to draw conclusions from the results of the attack regarding the morbidity and mortality associated with nerve agents. The lack of clinical data means that much of our knowledge of treatment of nerve agent exposure relies on experimental data and on clinical experience treating organophosphate exposures.

The structure and biologic action of nerve agents is similar to organophosphates, commonly used as insecticides. Nerve agents are clear and usually colorless liquids at room temperature and can be dispersed as either a vapor or a liquid. The four G-agents are odorless and more volatile than VX. GB (sarin) has the greatest degree of volatility—similar to that of water. VX is a persistent substance, commonly found in an oily state, which allows for greater stability on surfaces. In either liquid or vapor phase, they are able to penetrate both clothing and skin [2,3].

Mechanism of action

Nerve agents are organophosphorous cholinesterase inhibitors, which inhibit tyrylcholinesterase in the plasma, acetylcholinesterase on the red cell, and acetylcholinesterase at cholinergic receptor sites in the tissues. This leads to acetylcholine accumulation and binding to the cholinergic receptor site (Fig. 1). Acetylcholine continues to stimulate the affected organ

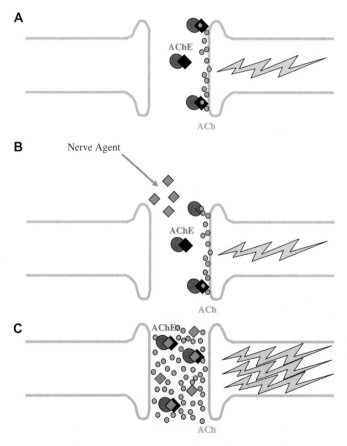

Fig. 1. Mechanism of action of nerve agent poisoning. (*A*) Normal neuronal signal conduction. (*B*) The victim is exposed to nerve agent. (*C*) The resulting accumulation of acetylcholine leading to nerve over stimulation. A similar effect will be seen at neuron–muscular and neuron–glandular junctions.

producing various symptoms. If measured after exposure, the red cell enzyme is a more sensitive indicator of tissue enzyme activity. During recovery, however, plasma enzyme is a more accurate reflection of tissue enzyme. It should be emphasized that in a mass casualty event these tests are unnecessary and time wasting and that the diagnosis is made based on clinical signs and symptoms.

After being inhaled, the agent rapidly crosses the alveolar interstitial space into the bloodstream. Although nerve agents are able to penetrate the skin, reaching the bloodstream this way takes more time and therefore exposure by this route is associated with delayed onset of symptoms. Symptoms of vapor inhalation have an onset of seconds to minutes compared with minutes to hours when exposure is through the skin. Poisoning may also occur through ingestion of the agent through the gastrointestinal tract.

Clinical diagnosis

Nerve agents induce numerous effects throughout the body with the ultimate effect and speed of onset dependent on the size of the droplet and the method by which it entered the body. Any organ with cholinergic receptors is a potential site of action for nerve agents; including the central nervous system, exocrine glands, smooth and skeletal muscle, cranial efferents, and ganglionic afferents. Clinically nerve agents exert their effects on the airway, eyes, nose, gastrointestinal tract, skeletal muscles, central nervous system, and skin.

Respiratory distress will be the most common and debilitating presenting symptom. The patient's airway will be compromised by both increased secretions and bronchoconstriction. Copious rhinorrhea will also exacerbate the patient's respiratory status. The victim's eyes will be injected and miosis will be present. Vision will commonly be blurred and painful. Profuse sweating unrelated to the environment will occur. Increased gastrointestinal motility is characteristic, with nausea, vomiting, diarrhea, and cramps. The muscles will demonstrate fasiculations, twitching, and weakness. Central nervous system effects are dose dependent. At small doses these may include difficulty thinking and impaired judgment. In large exposures the central nervous system symptoms may include loss of consciousness, seizures, and apnea.

Cardiovascular changes may present as either increased or decreased heart rate secondary to either anxiety or vagal involvement. Heart block may also occur. Blood pressure is commonly within normal limits until terminal decline. High levels of exposure may have a rapid onset and not allow time for the low and moderate exposure symptoms. These high-dose exposures may manifest as rapid loss of consciousness and possible seizures. Death from apnea results after respiratory muscle paralysis and respiratory center depression of the central nervous system.

Treatment

Antidotes for nerve agent poisoning are atropine and pralidoxime chloride (2-PAM). These may be given at a health care facility or self-administered with an auto-injector.

Atropine
Initial dose. Adults: 2 to 6 mg intravenously (IV) or intramuscularly (IM). Infants (0–2 years): 0.05 mg/kg IM. Pediatric: 1 to 4 mg IM.

Repeat doses. Adults: repeat in 2-mg doses until resolution of symptoms. Infants: 0.02 to 0.05 mg/kg IV. Pediatric: up to 6 mg in 2-mg doses.

2-PAM
Dose. Adults: 600 to 1800 mg IM or slow IV. Infants/pediatrics: 15 to 25 mg/kg IM or slow IV.
The patient should be re-evaluated every 3 to 5 minutes until secretions decrease and breathing becomes easier. If the patient is experiencing significant respiratory distress, the patient should be intubated. All severely injured patients should receive a benzodiazepine.

Diazepam
Dose. Adults: 5 to 10 mg slow IV. Infants/pediatric: 0.2 to 0.5 mg/kg slow IV.
Alternatively an equivalent dose of either lorazepam or midazolam may be administered. These will raise the seizure threshold and may prevent secondary anoxic brain injury in the case of a large exposure.

Outcome. Outcome data regarding nerve agent exposure is lacking. Most large-scale exposures have occurred in areas without modern medical facilities. It seems that following an exposure to sarin, most successfully treated casualties will be breathing spontaneously within 3 to 4 hours. With more persistent agents such as VX, this may take much longer. Complications such as anoxic brain injury will significantly affect this outcome. Neurologic symptoms following high-or low-dose exposure to nerve agents may persist for weeks; these symptoms, if they do occur, may include difficulty concentrating and sleeping, depression, nightmares, and impaired judgment [4]. Long-term complications may also affect the cardiovascular system as a result of damage to the heart occurring from hypoxemia as well as from arrhythmias at the time of acute poisoning.

Personal protection and decontamination

Principles of decontamination

All patients arriving at the hospital following a chemical agent exposure must be decontaminated before being allowed into the facility. The purpose of this decontamination is threefold. It will protect the patient from continued injury due to residual agent on his clothes and skin; it will protect the health care providers from injury due to this residual agent, and importantly, it will protect the facility itself and allow it to continue to function for the benefit of all the casualties.

Wet decontamination is the method of choice in a mass casualty scenario and is achieved by removing the casualty's clothing and washing the victim with water. This will be made more effective by adding a mild soap or bleach solution. Such a simple strategy will remove 95% of the agent and is appropriate for all agents. Patients who are incapacitated and/or ventilated will have to be decontaminated by specially trained and protected personnel. These personnel will need to be equal and trained in the use of personal protective equipment. A proposed decontamination scheme is presented in Fig. 2.

Personal protection

The most important items of personal protection are a hooded protective mask and protective clothing. Nonbreathable clothing provides protection against most molecules including water, vapor, and air. This provides a physical barrier not only from entrance but also from escape, which unfortunately places the individual at risk for heat injury. A two-part breathable clothing item is the military's choice and is known as the battledress overgarment. It is composed of two layers: a charcoal-impregnated inner layer that is capable of absorbing chemical vapors, liquid and biologic agents, toxins, and radioactive alpha and beta particles; and a tightly woven outer layer. Completing the protection includes protective rubber gloves and shoe covers.

Hospital organization for a nerve agent event

Planning

The unique requirements of a chemical event and the need for patient decontamination mean that a specific plan must be in place rather than a generic hospital emergency plan. Such a plan is a mission for the entire hospital and will require the mobilization of all hospital resources rather than only the emergency medicine department. A plan is only effective if the people involved in implementing it are aware of the plan or at least of its broad outline. Because dealing with such an event will require involvement of the entire institution, the principles of the response plan will have to be widely disseminated.

Training

Recognition of the specific syndromes of chemical exposure will require education of the clinical staff in advance. The support staff involved in

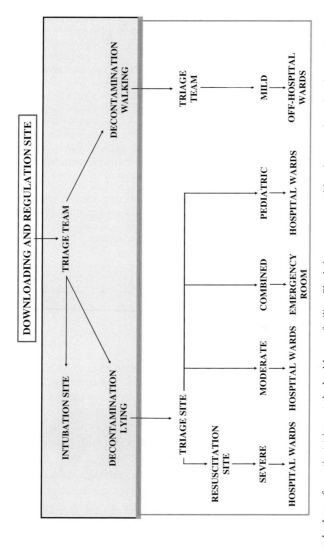

Fig. 2. A proposed scheme for patient triage at the health care facility. Shaded areas are considered contaminated and providers in these areas will require personal protection.

a chemical event will also require training in their roles: patient decontamination, security, assistance with patient ventilation by AMBU bag, or just transport of patients through the hospital. Ideally drills will be administered regularly to ensure the entire hospital is aware and understands each other's roles and responsibilities.

Logistics

Any mass casualty event will place a major strain on hospital resources. A chemical event will do so to an even greater extent because of its specific requirements. Particularly important will be: decontamination facility, drugs, patient care support systems, and personnel.

Decontamination facility

This is essential both to protect the patients from further injury due to residual agent on their skin and clothes and to protect the health care facility. Even if the local disaster plan is designed for decontamination at the scene of exposure, the hospital should anticipate a proportion of the casualties arriving untreated. The decontamination facility will need to be located outside the hospital in an adjacent area. The staff performing the decontamination will need protective garments.

Drugs

The hospital will need to stock adequate supplies of the specific antidotes for nerve agents. The amounts stocked will have to be based on the expected number of casualties.

Patient care support systems

All moderately to severely injured patients will require IV access. A significant number of patients may require ventilator support. Because the hospital may not have enough ventilators and ICU beds available, alternative plans should be worked out in advance.

Personnel

A chemical mass casualty event will require the mobilization of the hospital's entire resources. Although medical staff will probably be sufficient to deal with a mass casualty event, there will undoubtedly be a need for additional personnel in supporting functions. Security will be a major concern. It will be necessary to close the hospital to anyone trying to get in without going through the decontamination area first. Specifically trained teams will need to manage decontamination. These people do not need to be medical personnel. They do, however, need to be trained in the use of protective clothing and the principles of decontamination. Patient transport personnel will be important as well. Large numbers of wounded must be expected and they will not be able to walk. Personnel will need to be identified whose responsibility will be the transport of patients between treatment sites.

The anesthesiologist in a chemical event

Treatment of the chemically injured patient will not end in the emergency room. An unpredictable number will require anesthesia and critical care services. Anesthesiologists have proven to be a critical resource during other types of mass casualty events and can be expected to play a leading role during a mass chemical exposure with nerve agent [5]. The nature of a chemical event is that these patients will arrive within a period of hours necessitating a rapid expansion of ICU resources. Again advance planning for surge capacity is critical and this capacity will be required for an extended period as patients suffer from secondary complications of respiratory failure and possible anoxic brain injury.

Need for airway management

The mass casualty scenarios outlined will lead to a significantly increased requirement for mechanical ventilation. Before initiation of mechanical ventilation, thought will have to be given to the issue of airway control. Mass casualty nerve agent intoxication will present unique airway management challenges in several respects. In a typical hospital scenario, patients commonly require airway manipulation in the operating room and less frequently in the ICU or emergency room. Occasionally patients will deteriorate on other hospital floors and require an emergency airway intervention in another location.

In a mass casualty scenario involving use of nerve agents, we can expect that many more patients will need airway interventions outside the operating room. These patients will be sicker then those typically managed in the operating room and require more emergent management. These patients will present with respiratory failure exacerbated by bronchoconstriction and copious secretions. Many patients will be vomiting due to the gastrointestinal effects of the nerve agent. Most will be agitated and many will have an altered level of consciousness due to the effects of the agent. Patients who have had a delayed evacuation to the sight of medical care may already be suffering from the secondary effects of anoxic brain injury. These patients will present significant challenges in obtaining and protecting a viable airway.

Another unique aspect to mass casualty incidents involving chemical agents is the risk of exposure to the agent during airway manipulation. There is little data regarding this. Personnel are at risk from the clothing of undecontaminated patients. Planning for these scenarios will require consideration of personal protection for health care workers working in the decontamination area to minimize these risks. Once the patient has been decontaminated and is in the clean area of the hospital, inhaled agents will likely have been absorbed and do not present further risk to the health care provider. At this point standard airway precautions should suffice. Standardizing an institution's approach to airway management is also a key component in reducing risk to both health care worker and patient.

How should the airway be managed?

Endotracheal intubation has long been the gold standard of airway management, providing a secure airway and allowing positive pressure ventilation without air leak. In recent years alternative methods of securing the airway such as the laryngeal mask airway and various types of ventilating airways have been advocated for short-term management of the airway in both the perioperative setting and in situations requiring emergent airway management [6–8]. In the ICU, noninvasive ventilation using a tightly fitting face mask has gained favor in various clinical scenarios including acute respiratory failure [9]. Unfortunately none of these are practical alternatives in a mass casualty scenario involving chemical injuries.

Exposure risks require that the method of securing patient's airways minimize the risk to health care workers. The feasibility of using the laryngeal mask airway in emergent situations has been demonstrated, and in cases whereby health care workers are required to wear protective garments, they may actually shorten the time to obtaining airway control [10,11]. The laryngeal mask airway however provides an effective seal only up to pressures of 20 cm H_2O. These pressures will often be inadequate when ventilating patients who have severe bronchospasm. The resulting air leak will result in ineffective ventilation. Similar problems limit the use of noninvasive ventilation using a face mask. This is a resource-intensive mode because it requires considerable patient coaching to tolerate the tightly fitting mask and positive pressure ventilation. Although no method of controlling the airway provides perfect protection from aspiration of oral or gastric secretions, noninvasive ventilation will likely be the least effective protection.

Endotracheal intubation will therefore be the safest and most effective way of controlling the airway in a mass casualty scenario. Endotracheal intubation using full chemical protective gear is feasible although time to achieving control of the airway while encumbered in such a suit may be longer. This is not surprising because similar advanced resuscitative techniques such as placement of intraosseous access have been shown to take up to 50% more time to completion while the operator is wearing protective gear [12]. Advance training for the providers who are expected to manage the airway in a disaster will shorten these times [13,14]. Recently, use of simulators has been shown to reduce time to completion of the procedures and to improve provider comfort with attempting airway manipulation while wearing full chemical protection [15]. Alternative methods of airway control should be reserved for the rare case of unexpected difficult intubation whereby they may be life saving [16]. They should be replaced at the earliest possible time using fiberoptic bronchoscopy. Once the airway has been secured, proper placement should be confirmed, both by auscultation and by use of a disposable CO_2 detector.

Summary

Nerve agents are the subject of much mythology. They are well characterized and the treatment is straight forward. The logistical issues around treating a mass casualty event may however be daunting and require advance planning and preparation. Anesthesiologists will be a critical hospital resource in the event of a nerve agent incident and need to become familiar with the pathophysiology and treatment of nerve agent victims.

References

[1] Kales SN, Christiani DC. Acute chemical emergencies. N Engl J Med 2004;350(8):800–8.

[2] Available at: http://www.bt.cdc.gov/agent/nerve/. Accessed January 2007.

[3] Army of the United States. Textbook of military medicine; medical aspects of chemical and biological warfare. Available at: http://www.bordeninstitute.army.mil/cwbw/default_index.htm. Accessed January 2007.

[4] Morita H, Yanagisawa N, Nakajima T, et al. Sarin poisoning in Matsumoto, Japan. Lancet 1995;346(8970):290–3.

[5] Shamir MY, Weiss YG, Willner D, et al. Multiple casualty terror events: the anesthesiologist's perspective. Anesth Analg 2004;98(6):1746–52.

[6] Hagberg CA. Special devices and techniques. Anesthesiol Clin North America 2002;20(4):907–32.

[7] Dorges V, Wenzel V, Knacke P, et al. Comparison of different airway management strategies to ventilate apneic, nonpreoxygenated patients. Crit Care Med 2003;31(3):800–4.

[8] Idris AH, Gabrielli A. Advances in airway management. Emerg Med Clin North Am 2002;20(4):843–57, ix.

[9] Mehta S, Hill NS. Noninvasive ventilation. Am J Respir Crit Care Med 2001;163(2):540–77.

[10] Goldik Z, Bornstein J, Eden A, et al. Airway management by physicians wearing anti-chemical warfare gear: comparison between laryngeal mask airway and endotracheal intubation. Eur J Anaesthesiol 2002;19(3):166–9.

[11] Ben-Abraham R, Weinbroum AA. Laryngeal mask airway control versus endotracheal intubation by medical personnel wearing protective gear. Am J Emerg Med 2004;22(1):24–6.

[12] Ben-Abraham R, Gur I, Vater Y, et al. Intraosseous emergency access by physicians wearing full protective gear. Acad Emerg Med 2003;10(12):1407–10.

[13] Hendler I, Nahtomi O, Segal E, et al. The effect of full protective gear on intubation performance by hospital medical personnel. Mil Med 2000;165(4):272–4.

[14] Flaishon R, Sotman A, Ben-Abraham R, et al. Antichemical protective gear prolongs time to successful airway management: a randomized, crossover study in humans. Anesthesiology 2004;100(2):260–6.

[15] Berkenstadt H, Ziv A, Barsuk D, et al. The use of advanced simulation in the training of anesthesiologists to treat chemical warfare casualties. Anesth Analg 2003;96(6):1739–42.

[16] Practice guidelines for management of the difficult airway: an updated report by the American Society of Anesthesiologists Task Force on Management of the Difficult Airway. Anesthesiology 2003;98(5):1269–77.

**ELSEVIER
SAUNDERS**

Anesthesiology Clin
25 (2007) 201–208

**ANESTHESIOLOGY
CLINICS**

Index

Note: Page numbers of article titles are in **boldface** type.

Moving?

Make sure your subscription moves with you!

To notify us of your new address, find your **Clinics Account Number** (located on your mailing label above your name), and contact customer service at:

E-mail: elspcs@elsevier.com

800-654-2452 (subscribers in the U.S. & Canada)
407-345-4000 (subscribers outside of the U.S. & Canada)

Fax number: 407-363-9661

Elsevier Periodicals Customer Service
6277 Sea Harbor Drive
Orlando, FL 32887-4800

*To ensure uninterrupted delivery of your subscription, please notify us at least 4 weeks in advance of move.